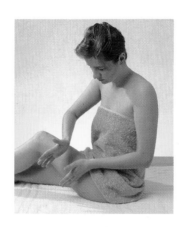

THE COMPLETE
MASSAGE
COURSE

To

Ros.

Lets have some fun!

love always.

Lisa
x

Christmas 2002.

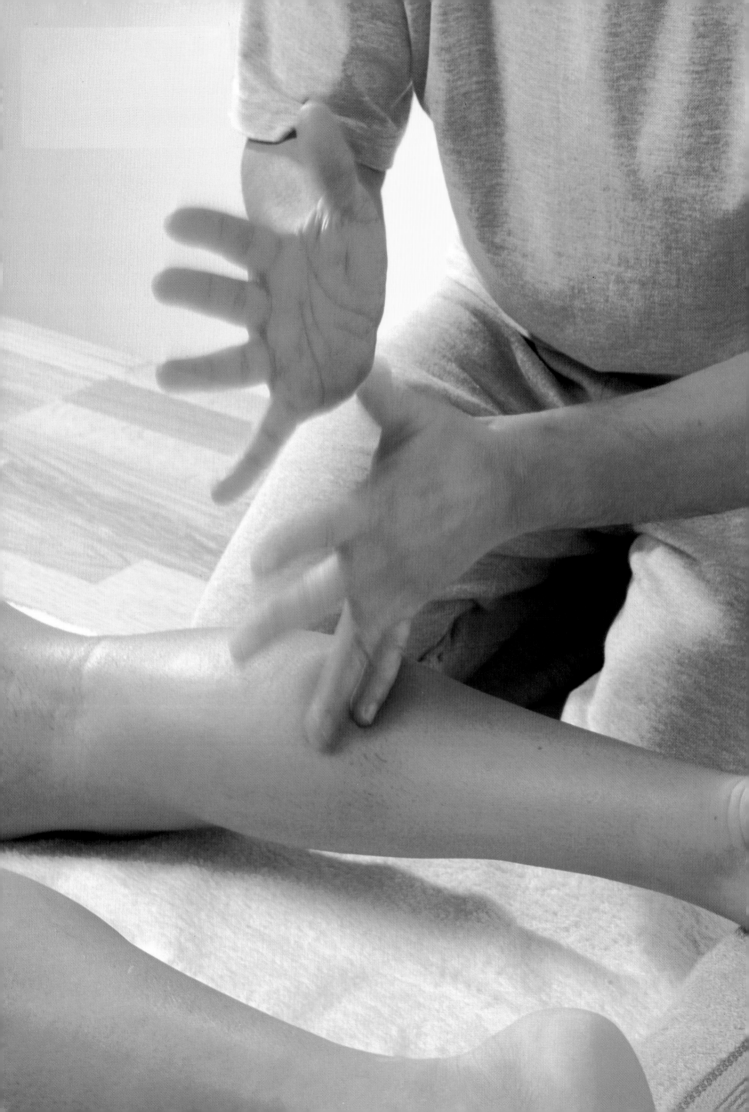

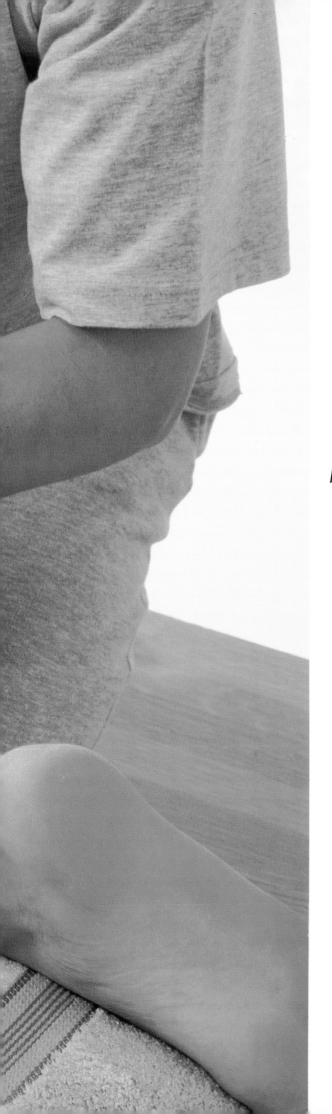

THE COMPLETE
MASSAGE
COURSE

MARIO-PAUL CASSAR

CHANCELLOR
PRESS

A QUANTUM BOOK

This edition published in 2000 by Chancellor Press
An imprint of Bounty Books, a division of
Octopus Publishing Group Ltd
2-4 Heron Quays
London
E14 4JP

ISBN 0-75370-366-1

QUMHGM

This book was produced by
Quantum Publishing
6 Blundell Street
London N7 9BH

Printed in Singapore by Star Standard Industries Pte Ltd

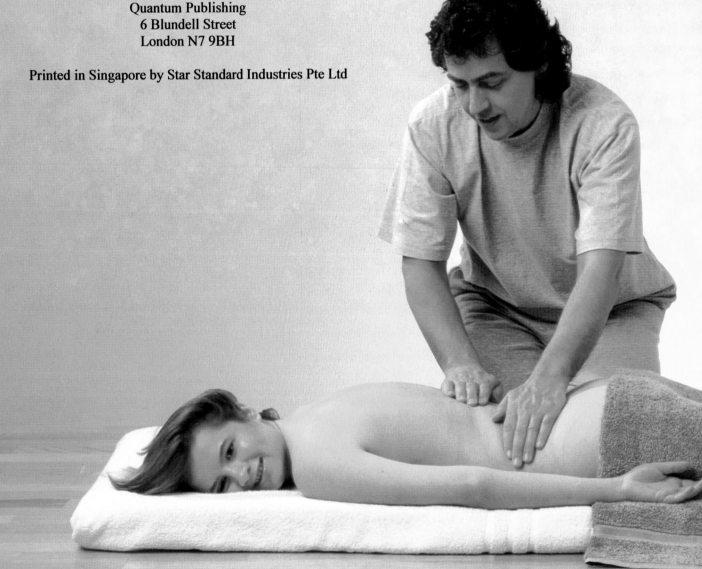

FOREWORD

· · · · · · · · · · · · · · · ·

T he practice of massage goes back thousands of years, but in its modern form it was first introduced in Europe in the early nineteenth century. Together with exercise, it formed a treatment regime for many conditions, including arthritis and rheumatism. Due to the fact that it was practised exclusively in hospitals in those early days it was looked upon with respect. As it gradually became more widely available, though, its application tended to become casual, and in some cases questionable, and it lost much of its credibility. Fortunately, in more recent times, massage has again become accepted for its therapeutic values. This may partly result from the increase in popularity of alternative and complementary medicine. However, there is still some way to go for it to achieve full public recognition and to regain the esteem it deserves. I hope that this book will help, albeit in a small way, to make this happen.

My aim in writing the book is to guide the reader through a number of massage techniques which are easy to master, safe to use and very effective. The step-by-step massage routines can be used on friends, family, colleagues and, in some cases, as self-administered treatment.

I have demonstrated the massage movements with the recipient either lying down on the floor or sitting on a chair to illustrate the feasibility of massage at home, in the office, and so on. The techniques can be easily adapted for use on a massage plinth and by a professional massage therapist. Using a plinth is generally more comfortable for the person doing the massage, but it is a matter of preference and availability.

For massage to be of benefit, the massage therapist must have a good understanding of its effects. To this end, I have included information on the physiological processes and objectives connected with the various techniques. I hope that this will also add to the interest and enjoyment of both the recipient and the giver.

The techniques I have shown illustrate the use of massage not only for relaxation but also as a treatment for conditions frequently encountered. This is not a claim for massage as a cure, but a way of demonstrating its therapeutic value and application, as an instrument of first aid or an adjunct to medical or other complementary treatment.

Writing this book reminded me of the start of my massage career. Many years ago I picked up a health magazine which was running a monthly feature of massage movements. I tried them out on friends and their reaction was very positive and encouraging. The subject fascinated me so much that I embarked on a number of courses on massage and bodywork, and eventually changed my career. It is, for me, very satisfying and exciting to think that the reader of this book, if he or she happens to be giving a massage for the first time, may experience the same enjoyment and fascination I did in my early days, and still do today.

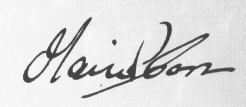

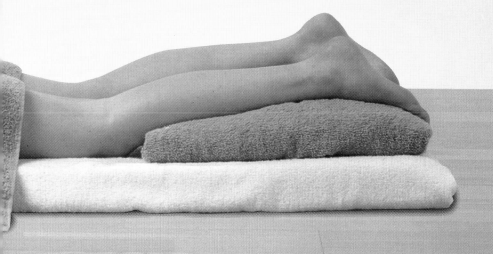

Contents

How to use this book

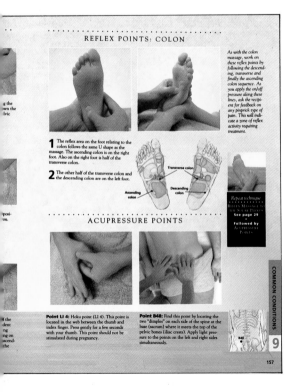

Reflex and acupressure features complement the massage techniques

Repeat techniques are explained earlier or later in the book. If you are doing a routine make sure that you include them in the correct places in the sequence

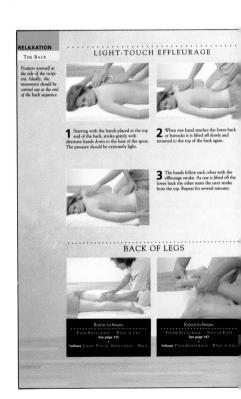

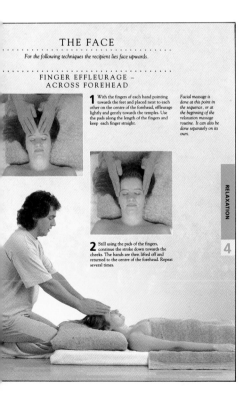

THE FACE

For the following techniques the recipient lies face upwards.

FINGER EFFLEURAGE –
ACROSS FOREHEAD

1 With the fingers of each hand pointing towards the feet and placed next to each other on the centre of the forehead, effleurage lightly and gently towards the temples. Use the pads along the length of the fingers and keep each finger straight.

Facial massage is done at this point in the sequence, or at the beginning of the relaxation massage routine. It can also be done separately on its own.

2 Still using the pads of the fingers, continue the stroke down towards the cheeks. The hands are then lifted off and returned to the centre of the forehead. Repeat several times.

RELAXATION

4

Routines indicate a suggested order for the techniques. These can be followed or adapted to suit personal preference

Introduction to each technique. It is important to read this before you do the technique

It is vital to read the "Take care not to" boxes, as these contain important safety information

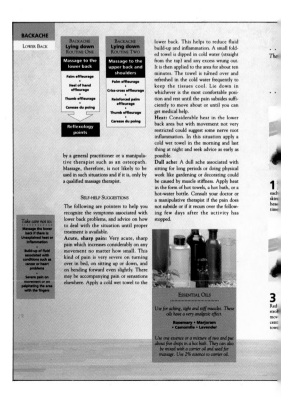

BACKACHE

LOWER BACK

BACKACHE
Lying down
ROUTINE ONE

Massage to the lower back

Palm effleurage

Heel of hand effleurage

Thumb effleurage

Caresse du poing

Reflexology points

BACKACHE
Lying down
ROUTINE TWO

Massage to the upper back and shoulders

Palm effleurage

Criss-cross effleurage

Reinforced palm effleurage

Thumb effleurage

Caresse du poing

by a general practitioner or a manipulative therapist such as an osteopath. Massage, therefore, is not likely to be used in such situations and if it is, only by a qualified massage therapist.

SELF-HELP SUGGESTIONS

The following are pointers to help you recognize the symptoms associated with lower back problems, and advice on how to deal with the situation until proper treatment is available.

Acute, sharp pain: Very acute, sharp pain which increases considerably on any movement no matter how small. This kind of pain is very severe on turning over in bed, on sitting up or down, and on bending forward even slightly. There may be accompanying pain or sensations elsewhere. Apply a cold wet towel to the

lower back. This helps to reduce fluid build-up and inflammation. A small folded towel is dipped in cold water (straight from the tap) and any excess wrung out. It is then applied to the area for about ten minutes. The towel is turned over and refreshed in the cold water frequently to keep the tissues cool. Lie down in whichever is the most comfortable position and rest until the pain subsides sufficiently to move about or until you can get medical help.

Heat: Considerable heat in the lower back area but with movement not very restricted could suggest some nerve root inflammation. In this situation apply a cold wet towel in the morning and last thing at night and seek advice as early as possible.

Dull ache: A dull ache associated with sitting for long periods or doing physical work like gardening or decorating could be caused by muscle stiffness. Apply heat in the form of hot towels, a hot bath, or a hot-water bottle. Consult your doctor or a manipulative therapist if the pain does not subside or if it recurs over the following few days after the activity has stopped.

Take care not to:
Massage the lower back if there is:
Unexplained heat or inflammation
Build-up of fluid associated with conditions such as cancer or heart problems
Severe pain on movement or on palpitating the area with the fingers

ESSENTIAL OILS

Use for aching, tight and stiff muscles. These oils have a very analgesic effect.

Rosemary • Marjoram • Camomile • Lavender

Use one essence or a mixture of two and put about five drops in a hot bath. They can also be mixed with a carrier oil and used for massage. Use 2% essence to carrier oil.

The

1
each
skin
head
time

3
Red
stro
mov
cent
towa

1

INTRODUCTION

INTRODUCTION

. . . .

Massage has probably existed as long as there have been human beings. It is a natural instinct to "rub away pain", which can be considered as the simplest form of massage.

Archaeological discoveries indicate that prehistoric people used ointments and herbs to rub their bodies. This is likely to have been intended to promote general well-being, and for protection from injury or infection. The potions would also have had a healing effect, especially if the "rubbing of the body" was done by a religious or medical healer.

Chinese literature records that massage was used for healing as far back as 3000 BC. The Chinese seem to have believed in "complete health", and massage, along with exercise, martial arts and meditation was included in all their health and fitness programmes.

Hindu writing dating from 1800 BC indicates that massage was used for weight reduction and to aid sleep, relaxation and combating fatigue. The Hindus were more interested in hygiene than health and so combined massage with bathing and shampooing.

Around 300 BC the Greeks started to make use of massage, coupling it with exercise as a regime for fitness. Soldiers were given regular massages to help ease pain and muscle fatigue during training, and also before and after tournaments. Greek ladies associated massage with bathing, and it became a fashionable part of their beauty regimes.

The Greek physician Herodicus (fifth century BC) professed to have had great success in prolonging lives with the combination of massage, herbs and oils. One of his pupils, Hippocrates, (the father of medicine who lived around 460–380 BC) followed suit and claimed he could improve joint function and increase muscle tone with massage. He also stated that the massage strokes should be carried out towards the heart rather than the feet. This was astonishing, since there was no knowledge of blood circulation at that time.

The Romans followed the Greeks' example in the use of massage. They went even further and built public baths available to rich and poor alike. Here they could have a leisurely soak in a communal hot bath, followed by a good rubdown with sweet-smelling oils.

Massage was valued not only for its beneficial effects on muscles but also for conditions such as headaches. Celus, a prominent Roman physician, who lived during the reign of Tiberius (42 BC–AD 37), claimed it even cured paralysis.

FROM THE RENAISSANCE ONWARDS

Books of the Renaissance period describe massage treatments, possibly because they became popular with royalty. In France, for example, physician Ambroise Pare (1517–90) was very sought after by the royal household for his massage treatments, and Mary Queen of Scots (1542–87) was also enthusiastic about it.

This Attic vase c.430 BC, shows a youth massaging the back of a friend.

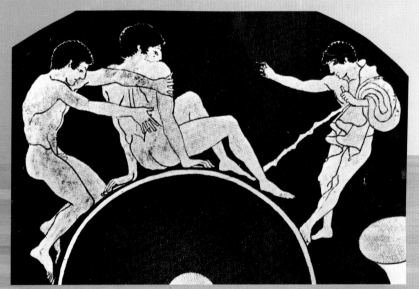

In the eighteenth century Captain James Cook was treated to a massage for his sciatic pain by a Polynesian family. He was so pleased with its benefits that he shared his experience in the writings of his journeys around the world.

In more modern times the word synonymous with massage in many people's minds is "Swedish". The technique it refers to was developed in Sweden in the late eighteenth century by a physician called Per Henrik Ling (1776–1839), who formulated the science of "gymnastics", which was a treatment combining massage and exercise. The massage part was later to be taken out of context and practised as Swedish massage.

In the UK, John Grosvenor (1742–1823), an English surgeon and professor of medicine at Oxford University, demonstrated the benefits of massage in relieving stiff joints, gout and rheumatism. Grosvenor, however, did not include exercise as part of his treatment; he was mostly interested in the healing of tissues and joints by the action of friction or rubbing. He claimed that this technique abolished the need to conduct operations in many diseases. Unlike other physicians, Grosvenor did not carry out the massage himself. He taught the techniques to women who were employed as nurse assistants.

DECLINE IN REPUTATION

By the nineteenth century the number of women in England offering massage had increased considerably. Originally they were trained by physicians, but due to increased demand, a number of massage schools opened up. This step into commercialism led to a lowering of teaching standards. The practice of massage was no longer governed by hospitals; it became available on a private basis. "Body shampooing" was at the same time being offered at Turkish baths. The outcome of all these changes was a rapid decline in the good reputation and credibility massage had previously enjoyed. The medical profession had every reason to look down upon dubious characters offering massage and advertising themselves as "rubbers" and "professors".

Surprisingly, Queen Victoria boosted the reputation of massage in the late 1880s. Per Henrik Ling, the Swedish physician, had founded the Central Gymnastics Institute of Berlin in 1813 and appointed Lars Gabriel Branting as his successor. One of Branting's students, Lady John Manners, Duchess of Rutland, wrote many articles about massage for "upper class" magazines , and arranged for Branting to treat Queen Victoria's rheumatic pains. The much publicized success of Branting's treatment by "gymnastics" (massage and exercises) created a new demand for the therapy. As this practice became more fashionable massage gained some respectability.

MASSAGE IN THE USA

Massage was introduced in the USA by, among others, George Henry Taylor (1821–96) and his brother Charles Fayette Taylor (1826–99). Both had travelled to Europe originally to study the Ling method. Another advocate of massage at the time was Dr S. Weir Mitchell of Philadelphia, Pennsylvania, and one of the earliest books on massage written in English was published in 1884 by Dr O. Gragham of Boston, Massachusetts.

During the First World War, massage was used in English hospitals to treat injuries. Its benefits were highlighted by Sir Robert Jones, director of the Special Military Surgery Hospital in London: "As a concomitant to surgical treatment, massage may be employed to alleviate pain, reduce oedema, assist circulation and promote the nutrition of tissues."

In modern times massage has taken many directions but it still forms the essence of relaxation and many other therapies. Its benefits have been well examined, proved and recorded throughout its history.

THE BENEFITS OF MASSAGE

The most immediate and most noticeable effect of massage is relaxation, which is why it is so commonly associated with reducing tension. But it is not always designed to relax. Sometimes it has an invigorating effect; at other times it is employed to help drain away congestion in tissues or to ease contracted muscles and spasms.

The general function of the body is enhanced when it is in a relaxed state. Massage, therefore, influences the whole body in many different ways. Some of its beneficial uses are: to increase the circulation to an area like a muscle or a joint; to reduce pain; to relax muscles; to relax the recipient; to increase the circulation away from an area and assist drainage of excess fluid; to introduce essential oils into the skin.

RELAXATION

It is very instinctive and natural to "stroke" someone if you want to make them feel better. Equally natural and involuntary is for the person receiving the stroking to relax. The process is likely to be a two-way emotional exchange. Receiving a massage gives the recipient a feeling of being cared for. Giving a massage may subconsciously impart the feeling of being accepted to the giver.

THE BODY'S NERVOUS SYSTEM

The body contains a system of nerves whose job it is to monitor its own internal and the external environment. Information, in the form of electrical impulses, travels along the nerves to the brain which, in turn, stimulates the body to adapt to any changes. For example, if the external environment is cold the body will adjust by shivering to produce heat and by shutting off the blood supply to the skin to cut down further heat loss.

This very complex system is called the autonomic nervous system. It is responsible, on an unconscious level, for all bodily functions and for maintaining the body at optimum health, called homeostasis. If the external or internal environment spells "danger" then the system responds by raising the blood pressure, preparing the muscles for work and increasing the breathing rate. When the "danger" is over, the system causes the muscles to relax, the breathing to slow down and the blood pressure to lower.

Thus relaxing the body and the mind stimulates the autonomic nervous system towards achieving optimum health by enhancing bodily functions. Digestion improves, blood pressure reduces, pain-killing chemicals are released, hormone action is balanced. Massage can have a great influence on the autonomic nervous system through its soothing effect on the nerve endings in the skin and the calming down of the whole body.

MASSAGING MUSCLES

Most massage involves the direct contact of hands on skin. The massage affects structures lower down. Underneath the skin is a layer of tissue containing nerves, arteries, veins, lymph vessels and varying amounts of water and fat. These latter two give the skin its quality and appearance, and are responsible for the great variety of external shapes. The next layer down is the muscle layer which covers almost the whole body. In some areas there are three layers of muscle; in others only one or two. All the layers are worked on and influenced by massage.

Muscles can take a fair amount of pressure and stretching. It is therefore safe to massage all areas covered by muscle as long as the pressure is acceptable to the recipient. Areas like the abdomen

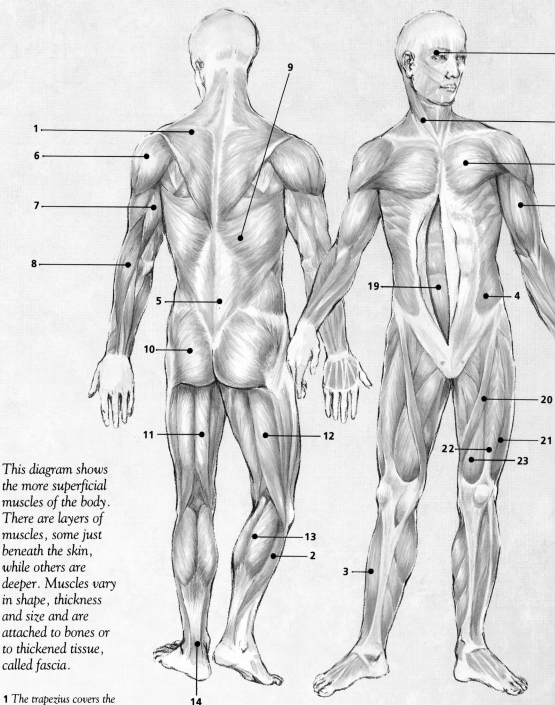

This diagram shows the more superficial muscles of the body. There are layers of muscles, some just beneath the skin, while others are deeper. Muscles vary in shape, thickness and size and are attached to bones or to thickened tissue, called fascia.

1 The trapezius covers the shoulder blade, the upper back and the back of the neck. It helps to rotate and lift up the shoulder blade and to bend the head backwards and to the side. **2** Underneath and further down the leg to the gastrocnemius is the soleus muscle which attaches to the achilles tendon and, with the gastrocnemius, helps to point the toes. **3** The most prominent muscle at the front of the lower leg is the tibialis anterior which attaches to the bones of the foot and helps to bend it upwards. **4** The internal and external oblique muscles run diagonally to the rectus abdominus. They work in pairs, left and

right, to bend the trunk forwards and to the side. **5** This area of the back is made up of layers of fascia (a strong type of tissue). **6** The deltoid muscle covers the shoulder joint. It raises and rotates the arm. **7** The triceps muscle joins the shoulder to the elbow and contracts to extend the forearm. **8** The brachioradialis muscle helps to turn the palm of the hand upwards. **9** Latissimus dorsi is a large muscle which connects the backbone to the humerus of the arm. **10** Gluteus maximus is the large muscle of the

buttock. It extends and rotates the thigh around the hip joint and also raises the trunk of the body from a stooping position. **11** Semitendinosus is a hamstring muscle which runs from the pelvis to the tibia below the knee. **12** Biceps femoris is one of the three hamstring muscles of the thigh which flex the knee and rotate it outwards. **13** The gastrocnemius muscle has two parts which together form nearly all of the calf. **14** The tendocalcaneus, or Achilles tendon, is the strongest tendon in the body and

connects the calf muscles to the ankle. **15** Orbicularis oculi lies in the orbit of the eye and surrounds it. This muscle closes the eyelid, wrinkles the forehead and squeezes tears into the eye. **16** The sternomastoid muscle runs down the side of the neck and stands out when it contracts. It either inclines the head towards the shoulder of the same side or rotates it towards the other side. **17** Pectoralis major is the large shoulder muscle which lies across the chest. It can either draw the arm forward or rotate it. **18** Biceps brachii runs

from the shoulder to the ulna in the forearm. It bends the arm at the elbow and helps to turn the palm upwards. **19** The two rectus abdominis muscles run down the front of the abdomen and bend the trunk of the body forward or to the side. **20** Sartorius is the longest muscle in the body, extending from the pelvis to the tibia. It rotates the thigh or raises it up to the abdomen, and also helps to bend the knee. **21** Vastus lateralis runs down the outside of the thigh. The fourth part of the quadriceps muscle, the vastus intermedius, lies between the vastus lateralis and medialis below the rectus femoris. **22** Rectus femoris is a long straight muscle at the front of the thigh which helps to raise the leg from the hip. Together with the three vastus muscles, it forms the quadriceps. The powerful group of muscles straightens out the leg and locks it in position when standing. **23** Vastus medialis runs down the inside of the thigh.

and neck need careful treatment, and bony areas should be avoided, as pressure on them can cause pain. Massage affects muscles in many ways. It increases the local circulation, helps to get rid of waste products in the tissues, reduces spasm and tension, and tones up muscle tissue.

BLOOD CIRCULATION

In a normal adult 5 litres (10 pints) of blood circulates and supplies every tissue and organ. The heart circulates 7000 litres (1539 gallons) of blood every day, pumping it first into the large arteries and then into smaller vessels called arterioles and capillaries. Continuous with the capillaries are small venules which carry the blood into larger veins and back to the heart. Having first visited the lungs for its oxygen to be replenished, the blood is pumped out again.

The heart exerts sufficient pressure to push the blood along the arteries, but by the time it arrives in the veins the pressure is reduced considerably and the blood requires the compressing action of muscles to help it along. The movements of massage help to push blood along the veins. Some strokes also improve the circulation along the arterioles and capillaries to areas like skin, hands and the feet.

Enhancing the general circulation is perhaps the most important effect of massage after that of relaxation.

LYMPH

Lymph is a fluid which is distributed throughout the body with the blood. As the blood passes through the very tiny capillaries the lymph seeps out, taking with it oxygen and nutrients. In the tissue spaces it surrounds every cell and supplies it with nourishment. On its return to the heart lymph picks up the by-products of cell function, waste products, viruses and bacteria and takes them through a separate system of vessels to the blood, called lymphatic vessels. These lead to filters called lymph nodes, where the lymph is treated and filtered before returning to the heart.

Lymph also relies on the action of the deep muscles to create compression and move it along its vessels. However, in the layer just below the skin the lymph fluid has to find its own drainage, as very little muscle action exists there. If there is any blockage along the way, or if too much fluid is produced, lymph tends to accumulate creating swelling, known as oedema. Very light massage strokes help to drain lymph fluid and so reduce oedema.

Conditions which benefit from massage
. . . .

The physiological effects of massage point to a number of conditions where massage can be beneficial. These include reduced peripheral circulation, lymphatic congestion, muscle spasms, tension and anxious states, flaccid musculature and backache. Some of these, like tension headache, are fairly uncomplicated to deal with. Others can also be helped by massage but within certain guidelines. More serious conditions may require professional help. Every condition can have complications: anxiety may result from underlying emotional problems; impaired circulation can be caused by heart failure; arthritis may be caused by mechanical and nutritional imbalances.

Conditions in which massage may be harmful
. . . .

While there is a lot to be gained from massage it may be harmful in some circumstances. It is inadvisable for the lay person at least to use massage in the following cases: cancer and associated conditions, like lymphoedema; heart and circulatory problems including left heart failure, thrombosis, migraine, varicose veins; inflammation of any bone, tissue or organ, such as rheumatoid arthritis, appendicitis, gastritis, pancreatitis, meningitis; some conditions involving the nervous system, like epilepsy.

MASSAGE OILS

. . . .

Massage oils facilitate the movement of the hands over skin by preventing friction, moisturize and soften the skin and, if they contain essential oils, enhance the therapeutic value of massage. Essential oils are extracts of herbs, spices, flowers, leaves, tree bark and resin, seeds, bulbs (garlic), dried flower buds (clove oil), and rinds of citrus fruits.

Essences have a long history of use and are mentioned in many ancient books including *Nei Ching* or *Yellow Emperor's Classic of Internal Medicine* written around the fourth century BC, and in the writings of the renowned Arab physician Abu Ali Ibn Sina (also known as Avicenna) who lived in the period AD 980–1037. These ancient records show that essences of flowers, plants and herbs had many uses and were administered in a number of ways, from massage oils to balms, medicinal cakes, suppositories, powders and pills. Their application included the treatment of war wounds suffered by gladiators and the fumigation of dead bodies. Throughout history they have been used as cosmetics, perfumes, insecticides, antiseptics, and even against epidemic infections like the plague of the seventeenth century.

In more recent times they were rediscovered by a French chemist, René Maurice Gattefossé, in the 1920s. At the time Gattefossé was researching the antiseptic properties of naturally extracted essential oils over those produced chemically. On one occasion, while working in the laboratory, he burnt his hand badly and plunged it into the nearest jar of liquid which happened to be lavender oil. To his amazement the hand healed within 48 hours. This rapid healing, together with the absence of any scars, inspired Gattefossé to research further into other properties of essential oils. The scientific values and medicinal properties of the oils were subsequently recorded in detail by Gattefossé, and Aromathérapie (as it was referred to by Gattefossé) was born. It is still practised in France by the medical profession.

CONSTITUENTS

The essences contain naturally occurring chemical compounds such as hydrocarbons (terpenes) and oxygenated compounds like alcohols, esters, ketones and phenols which give them their therapeutic properties. They can influence the body on both physical and emotional levels. Each essential oil has a number of properties. For example, camomile can be used as an antiseptic as well as an anti-inflammatory, to aid digestion or for relaxation.

As the oils are very volatile and evaporate quickly they are easily introduced into the body by inhalation through the nose. The sense of smell occurs via the olfactory nerve which goes direct from the nose to the brain. This very short pathway leads to immediate registration of any smell and a rapid reaction by the body. In addition, inhalation of the oils results in some molecules travelling to the lungs, where they are picked up by the circulation to be distributed throughout the body. Examples of these quick reaction inhalation pathways are demonstrated by the physical and mental effects resulting from glue-sniffing, nicotine and even anaesthetics. Another example, but more pleasant, is that of saliva being triggered in the mouth by the odour of freshly cooked food.

APPLICATION

One way of introducing essential oils into the body is by means of massage. They are first mixed with a "carrier oil". A vegetable oil is most commonly used, and is preferable to the liquid paraffin oil used

1

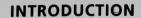

in some commercial baby oils. The aromatherapy oils are then massaged into the skin, to be absorbed and taken up by the lymphatic and vascular circulations. This idea of introducing therapeutic products into the body "transcutaneously" is very effective. We see its use in the orthodox field of medicine, an example of which is the application of sticking plasters in hormone replacement treatment. Another very effective method of encouraging absorption of the essential oils through the skin is to put them in a bath. Spread the drops of essences on the surface of the water, wait for them to spread out and then ease yourself in. The therapeutic value is gained not only through the absorption, but also from the aroma of the evaporating oils.

Applying the oils by way of a hot or cold compress has the added effect of cooling or warming a specific area of the body. This method is described fully in chapter 6.

The use of essential oils as a form of treatment can only be carried out by a qualified aromatherapist. However, oils can be used safely with massage to enhance its effects. They are available ready mixed, or you may want to mix your own essences with a carrier oil or in baths, as

EXAMPLES OF ESSENTIAL OILS SUITABLE FOR MASSAGE

Flowers
Camomile • Geranium • Jasmine • Lavender • Neroli • Rose

Herbs
Basil • Clary sage • Marjoram • Peppermint • Rosemary • Hyssop • Origanum • Thyme

Citrus
Bergamot • Grapefruit • Lemon

Resin
Frankincense • Myrrh

Seeds
Black pepper • Fennel

Leaves
Ti-tree • Petitgrain • Lemongrass • Melissa

Spices
Cinnamon • Cumin • Nutmeg

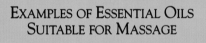

described above. Use only good quality essences produced by a reputable company. Use an average of three parts of essential oil to 100 parts of the carrier oil when mixing a massage oil. Use an average of five drops of essential oils in a bath or for a compress. For babies and children use only one or two drops (see chapter 8). You can mix two or three essences together as long as the total amount of three per cent remains the same. The use of essential oils can be very interesting provided you follow these guidelines. I would also recommend that you refer to one of the many books available on aromatherapy for further information.

PRECAUTIONS

Some oils can be toxic if used in large quantities or for extended periods, and can also lead to skin irritation if a person has allergic tendencies towards that particular oil. This is unlikely to happen with any of the oils included in this book.

However, if any reaction does occur or if any doubt exists, then it is best not to use them, and instead to apply an oil without any essences for the purpose of massage.

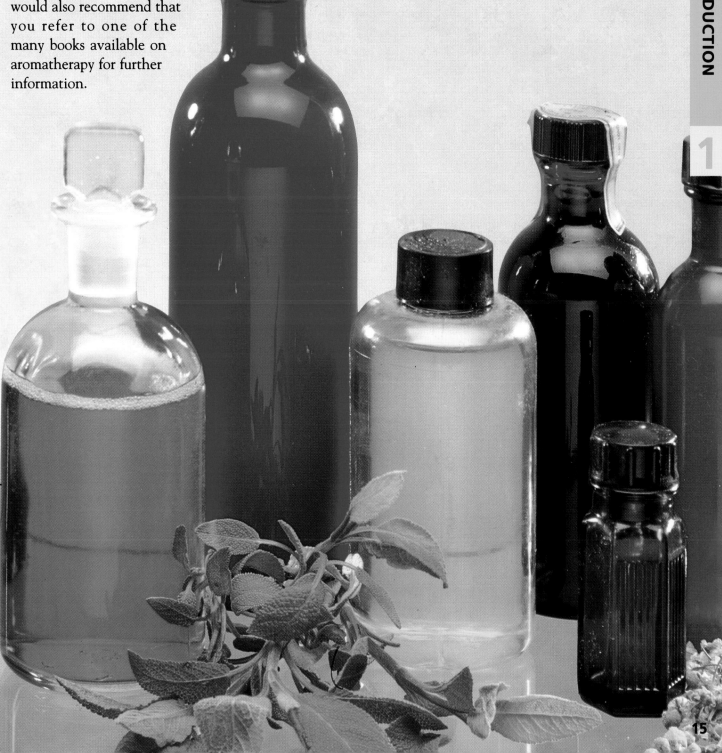

MASSAGE TECHNIQUES

Massage is both a science and an art. The science of massage is the effects it has on the tissues and on the body in general. The art of massage is knowing which strokes to apply and when. Together they constitute the techniques of massage.

Massage techniques have names like **effleurage, petrissage** and **thumb effleurage**. They are demonstrated in this book in step-by-step sequences. Later on in the book variations of these techniques are also included. They are my version of massage techniques; other massage practitioners may well interpret them differently.

A **stroke** or **movement** refers to the path or route the hands travel in a massage technique, which starts on one area of the body and ends either on another area or back at the same place. Massage strokes or movements are usually repeated several times, the number being dictated by what the giver and the recipient feel is sufficient. As a guide, each massage stroke is carried out at least six times or for a few minutes.

Rhythm is extremely important in massage as it sets the pace and determines what effect the technique is likely to have. With all massage techniques it is a good idea to check the recipient's reaction to the stroke, because what can be relaxing to one person may be uncomfortable to another.

Very slow: As a rule strokes are done very slowly for the purpose of relaxation. For example, a stroke from the lower end of the back up to the neck and down again would take about ten seconds.

Medium slow: Increasing the speed of the stroke stimulates the circulation to the area. Taking the back once more as an example, the movement described above would now take about five seconds.

Brisk: This can be used if you want to warm the muscles (and the recipient) in preparation for a sporting activity or generally for an invigorating effect. The speed of the movements is much faster. It may help you to compare this to rubbing your hands together when you want to warm them up.

Pressure needs to be constantly adjusted to the area being massaged. Applying hard pressure does not mean

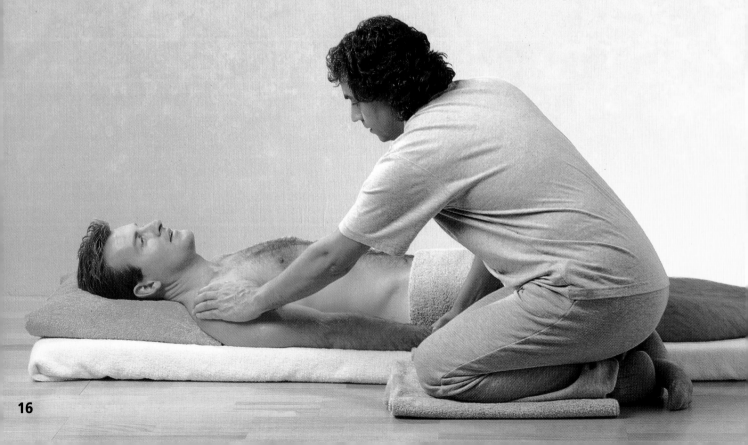

that the massage stroke is going to be more effective or more relaxing. The muscles, and the recipient, may not be ready for any heavy work. It could even have the opposite effect and cause a "protecting" tension within the muscle. It is advisable, therefore, to use the idea of encouraging rather than forcing muscles to relax. The pressure may be increased as long as the muscle is giving in to it and not resisting.

POSTURE

The techniques in this book can be used with the recipient lying on the floor or sitting on a chair. They may also be adapted for use on a massage plinth or table. Whatever the position of the recipient, the posture of the giver is very important. It must be adapted to ensure you are not creating any problems for yourself. Massaging someone on the floor can be tiring if you do not find a comfortable position while performing the movements. The illustrations depict positions

for the giver as well as the recipient. They are only guides, however, and can be altered if necessary. Whenever possible, use your body weight as part of the movement. This means you make less muscular effort, which makes it easier to massage, and saves you energy. It applies whether you massage with the recipient on the floor, on a plinth, or in a chair.

ROUTINE

While most people prefer the massage to start with the back, others opt for the face or feet to be massaged first. There may be times when only one area of the body is massaged, dictated by the need or preference of the recipient or by the time available. I have given massage routines in most chapters. These can be followed as indicated or adapted to suit personal preferences. If you create your own routine, bear in mind that, generally speaking, lighter strokes are carried out prior to heavier ones, and the relaxation routines can be of any form provided the rhythm is slow. Two routines I tend to favour are listed left.

WARMTH

Work in a warm room and cover the recipient throughout the massage so as to keep their body warm. Muscles which are cold will contract to maintain body heat and are therefore unable to relax.

CUSHIONS AND PILLOWS

No matter what the recipient's position, he or she must be comfortable, and the body adequately supported. Cushions can be used to support the back, the knees and the feet whenever necessary. Extra care is needed when the recipient is lying face down on the floor. Cushions or pillows may be required underneath the abdomen so that the back does not curve too much (this applies especially in people with a tendency towards excessive curvature of the small of the back).

ROUTINE A	ROUTINE B
Recipient lying supine (on back)	**Recipient lying prone (on front)**
Scalp • Face • Arms • Abdomen and chest • Legs	Upper back and shoulders • Neck • Lower back • Legs
Recipient lying prone (on front)	**Recipient lying supine (on back)**
Legs • Lower back • Upper back • Neck	Feet • Legs • Abdomen • Chest • Arms • Face

BASIC MASSAGE STROKES

Massage consists of strokes or techniques, each one having a particular effect, such as warming up the tissues, increasing circulation, and so on. Techniques also have variations such as double-handed or single-handed petrissage. They are carried out singularly, or in a routine to achieve an overall effect – general relaxation, reducing muscle spasm, preparing muscles for sport and so on. The following are some basic massage strokes, plus one or two variations.

EFFLEURAGE

"Effleurage" comes from the French word effleurer (to touch lightly). It is the name for the basic "stroking" technique in massage. It can be done very lightly and slowly, for a soothing effect, just as you would instinctively stroke a baby or a pet, or with a medium to heavy pressure at a faster speed, to increase circulation and relax muscles. When done with speed, effleurage is invigorating. There are many variations, such as palm effleurage, thumb effleurage, pick-up effleurage and caresse du poing (closed hand) effleurage which can be used selectively for particular areas of the body.

PALM EFFLEURAGE

An example of this technique is shown here being applied to the back. The movement starts and finishes at the lower back. Steps 1, 2, 3 and 4 follow the route the hands take to complete the effleurage movement. The initial pressure is no more than you would apply to stroke a cat or a dog. However, you need to add some weight to the stroke by leaning forwards with your body. This should still be an acceptable pressure to the recipient. The more you lean on (or push with your body weight if you are using a massage table) the more the pressure increases.

Take care not to:
- Apply heavy pressure on the spine itself, or over the bony parts of the shoulder blades
- Use the heel of the hand, but spread the pressure evenly all over the palm and fingers

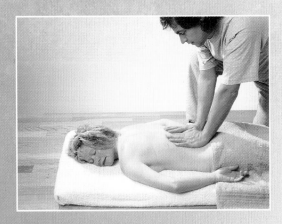 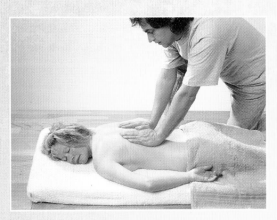

1 Starting at the base of the spine, effleurage upwards towards the head using the palms of both hands placed either side of the spine. Use very light pressure to start with and increase it gradually with each stroke, making sure it is always comfortable for the recipient.

2 Continue with the effleurage upwards over the middle back and rib cage.

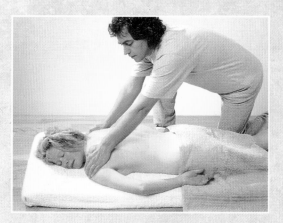

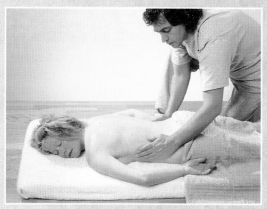

3 When the hands reach the top of the back continue the stroke over the shoulders. As you go round each shoulder cup your hands to cover the whole area and maintain some pressure.

4 Slide each hand down the outside of each arm and then on to the outside of the trunk to return to the lower back. Effleurage with the hands close to the spine for a few strokes, then follow this by a few strokes with the hands placed further away from the spine. Increase the pressure by shifting your body weight forwards and directly above the recipient.

· ·

THUMB EFFLEURAGE

This technique is used to massage more deeply into very tight muscles like those of the lower back. The thumbs are used alternately, each one applying a very short stroke over a small area of the muscle. The alternating strokes are repeated several times until a softening of the tissue is felt. The hands are then moved to a new position to work on another area of the same muscle. Pressure is slightly more than that of the palm effleurage – think of applying enough pressure to soften hard putty, plasticine or butter. If you find this difficult to imagine, think of reducing "knotted" muscle fibres. There may be times when the muscle tissue is not "tight" enough to need this technique. It is also possible to use this movement to increase the circulation to a small area like a finger or a toe. In this case the pressure is reduced.

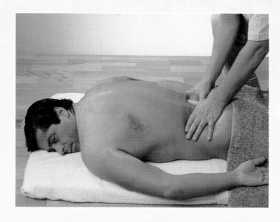

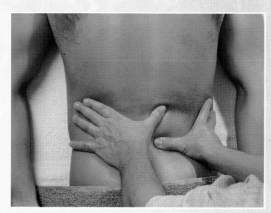

1 Place both hands so that the thumbs are on one side of the spine. Apply a very short stroke with one thumb following a fairly straight line towards the head. You may find it easier for the whole hand to move upwards towards the head with the thumb exerting most of the pressure.

2 The second thumb follows the same line towards the head and applies the same short stroke. It may be more comfortable for the pressure to be applied evenly with the whole hand until the thumbs get used to applying heavier pressure. The stroke is still very short and concentrates on a small area of muscle at a time.

CARESSE DU POING

This technique is used as an effleurage but exerting a fair amount of pressure. It is applied to areas like the small of the back or where the muscles are very tense. The technique is carried out by first closing each hand to make a fist and then using the back of the fingers to effleurage.

Take care not to:

Allow the fist to bend or twist in such a way as to exert pressure with the knuckles instead of the backs of the fingers

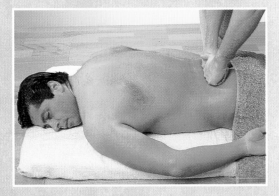

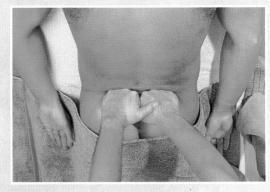

1 Place each hand, with the fingers curled into a fist, one on each side of the spine. The fist should be flat to the skin so that the knuckles do not dig in.

2 Keep the hands close to the spine as you effleurage upwards towards the head. Increase the pressure gradually as you lean forward to allow your body weight to transfer to your hands.

PETRISSAGE

Petrissage has been translated as "kneading", which is an appropriate description of the technique. Its effect is to soften and relax tense and tight muscles. This is achieved through the loosening of bunches of muscle fibres, which tend to harden and stick together if the muscle is overworked. It also increases the circulation through the muscle and helps to reduce toxins. The technique involves picking up a particular muscle or group of muscles and applying compression with both hands. Petrissage has many variations but here I am demonstrating one which uses the thumb of one hand and the fingers of the other to compress the muscles. In some areas it is easier to use the heel of the hand instead of the thumb. Having squeezed and twisted the muscle tissue it is released almost completely before it is lifted up again for a repeat compression.

Note: *Throughout the movement there is very little sliding of the fingers. The most suitable muscles for this technique are the larger groups like those of the leg, lower back, buttocks and arms.*

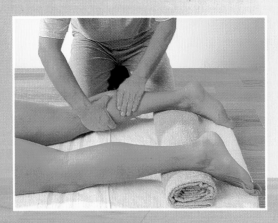

1 Place the fingers of each hand on the inside of the calf muscles and the thumbs on the outside. Your fingers should go round the muscles; the fingertips can apply a little extra pressure to help with grasping but without any digging into the tissues.

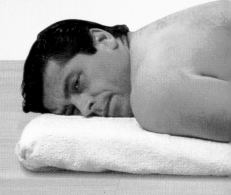

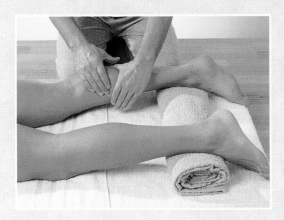

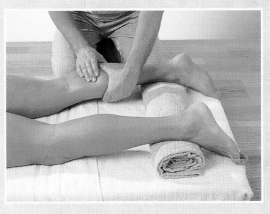

3 Move your hands around to cover as much of the calf muscles as possible. If your hands are too small or the muscle tissue is too large for your hands, the compression can be done between the fingers of one hand and the heel of the other.

2 Apply pressure between the two hands to compress and lift the muscles. Use the thumb of one hand against the fingers of the other hand. You can also twist the tissues gently between the two hands at the same time. Avoid pinching the skin.

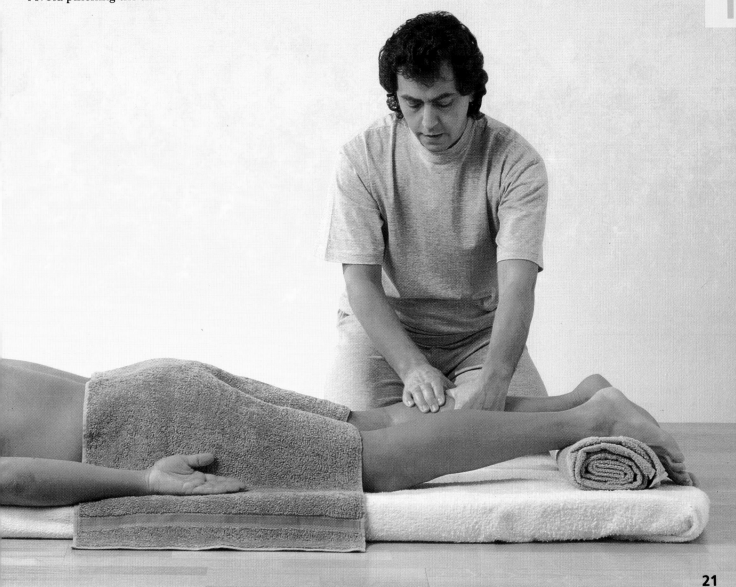

BASIC MASSAGE STROKES

Note: *It may help you to imagine that you are squeezing a hard-boiled egg with the shell removed, and not wanting to squash it. The technique is repeated several times until you can feel the loosening of the muscle.*

Take care not to:

The muscles in this area are likely to be tense, so do not apply too much or too sudden a pressure

•

Use effleurage techniques prior to, or as a substitute for kneading if the muscles are very tight

KNEADING

This technique is carried out with one hand and the action is more of a kneading action than that of the previous petrissage. The single-handed kneading achieves the same effect as the two-handed petrissage but it is mostly carried out on smaller muscles like the one at the top of the shoulder, the upper trapezius muscle. The compressing of the muscle is done with the heel of the hand and the fingers, except that the fingers have more of a supporting role rather than compressing. The pressure is increased gradually with each stroke.

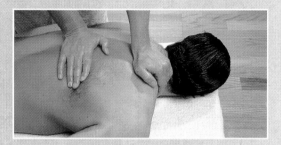 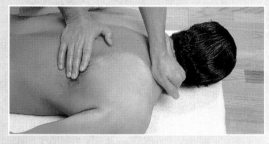

1 Work on the shoulder furthest away from you, first lifting up the muscle with the fingers. Do not press with the fingertips too much as this can be a tender area. The heel of the hand is placed lower down on the muscle in between the spine and the shoulder blade. Apply a compressing pressure on the muscle with the heel of the hand at the same time as sliding towards the top of the shoulder.

2 When the heel of the hand reaches the top of the muscle gently release the grip. Do not squeeze the skin at the end of the movement. Once the heel of the hand is returned to the starting position the fingers lift the muscle again for the stroke to be repeated.

PERCUSSIVE STROKES: LITTLE FINGER STRIKE

Percussive strokes increase the local circulation of the skin. They also stimulate the nerve endings, resulting in tiny muscular contractions. The overall effect is increased tone in the muscles (i.e. increased responsiveness of muscle to nerve impulses).
The little finger strike is also known as hacking. The little finger of each hand alternately applies a light percussive strike on the muscle tissue, with the hand bending from the wrist, and the pressure controlled and kept to a minimum.

Note: *It is not easy to judge when the tissues are toned up, so these alternating strokes are carried out for a few minutes only, or until the recipient feels it is time to stop.*

Take care not to:

Use percussive strokes on:

•

The spine or bony areas

•

Any strained, inflamed or tender tissue

•

On varicose veins

•

On the head, the chest, the abdomen or neck

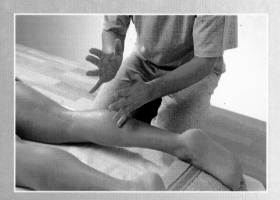 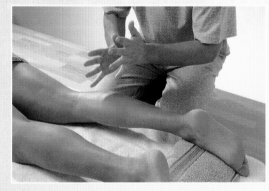

1 Place the hands above the area to be percussed, keeping the fingers straight and apart. With one of the hands, begin the stroke by hitting the tissues with the little finger as you bend the wrist. As the hand hits the tissues the fingers will cascade down on each other so that they are temporarily closed together.

2 Lift the hand up again to complete a flicking movement and at the same time bring down the second hand. Repeat the stroke with the hands alternating several times.

PERCUSSIVE STROKES: CUPPING

This is done with the hand in a cupped position, and sounds a bit like a horse's hoofs clip-clopping along. Cup the hands and imagine you are holding a table tennis ball in each hand with the palms turned downwards but without closing the fingers. Apply sufficient tapping pressure to stimulate the skin without causing any discomfort. The strokes are repeated for a minute or two or until the recipient feels that it is time to stop.

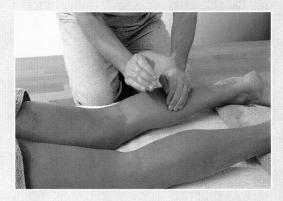 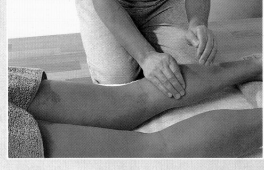

1 Position the hands so that they are above the area to be percussed. Carry out the movement with the wrist almost straight and the entire forearm moving up and down to percuss.

2 As the hand hits the tissues, immediately lift it up again, but unlike the finger percussion this is not done in a "flicking" manner. The second hand begins to come down as the first one is lifted up.

MASSAGE TO AID LYMPH DRAINAGE

The aim here is to assist the passage of lymph along the lymph vessels and reduce any oedema, or swelling, which may be present. The pace at which lymph moves naturally is very slow, and the massage to assist it matches this speed. Lymph drainage requires very light pressure to avoid compressing the vessels and restricting the free flow of the fluid. The stroke used is very light and slow effleurage, carried out towards the lymph nodes, which are located at key zones like the groin, the back of the knee and the armpit. The movement is more of a "dragging forwards" of the hands rather than that of applying pressure. The weight of the hand itself should be almost sufficient. Each stroke is repeated several times. An example is given below.

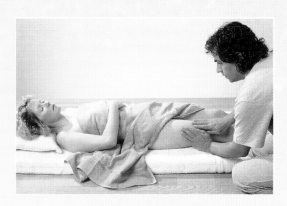 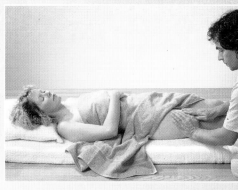

1 The thigh can be drained by effleuraging first the outer and then the inner areas. The hands work very close together, and contact is made with the whole hand. From the outer region move very slowly towards the inguinal nodes in the groin, taking about eight seconds to travel from the lower to the upper end of the thigh.

2 When you reach the groin return to the starting position to repeat the movement. Do this several more times but with the hands at the inner aspect of the thigh. Effleurage towards the groin area as in the previous stroke.

Take care not to:
....
Attempt massage for lymphatic drainage in conditions where there is:
Unexplained heat or inflammation
•
Swelling throughout the whole body associated with any condition like cancer or heart problems
•
Lymphoadenoma (tumour of lymphoid tissue)
•
Lymphoedema (oedema due to obstruction of lymphatics)
•
Breast cancer

ACUPRESSURE

The Chinese and Japanese developed the art and application of massage to localized specific areas of the body. Shiatsu and Acupressure are two examples of their treatments.

Balancing the energy to treat people physically has been a healing concept in China and Japan for thousands of years. The body's energies were mentioned in Japanese literature of the sixth century AD. Acupressure, which is older than acupuncture, was used by doctors in China, and later on by lay people, probably as far back as the fifth century BC. One story which may have heralded the research into "energy treatment" all those thousands of years ago describes how a soldier was hit by an arrow on his achilles tendon, just above the heel. Having had the arrow removed, he discovered that the arthritic condition he had previously suffered from had abated. Another possible explanation may have had a religious and cultural origin. The Chinese believed that for a person to go to heaven the body had to be buried intact. This created a dilemma for the physicians because they were not allowed to operate on it or dissect it. It is also said that doctors were only allowed to see their patients fully dressed.

This may have been the background to the development of the Chinese system of diagnosis and treatment. Diagnosis involved observing the patient's face, eyes, wrinkles, breath, tongue and voice, and assessing the strength and rhythms of the body's pulses. Treatment included light touch on specific points; acupuncture with needles; prescribing herbs, meditation, martial arts and exercises. Names given for treatments included Jin Shin Jitsu, Tsubo points, Shiatsu, and Acupressure.

ENERGY CHANNELS

The concept of energy fields defines twelve paths through the body, known as meridians. Each path passes through organs, skin surfaces, muscles, and so on. The energy known as Ki (vital life force) flowing through the body is said to be synonymous with cosmic energy en route to the earth, and vice-versa. People are therefore governed by the same energy laws that govern micro-organisms and the universe. This energy is constantly flowing and is responsible for constant change and balance (Yin and Yang, a spiral of change). Any interruption or excessive build-up of this energy through any of the pathways or meridians has an adverse effect on the body, resulting in disease, malfunction, emotional trauma, and so on. Feeling for the energy and balancing its flow constitutes the science and the art of all energy-based therapies, including that of acupuncture. Proof of the powerful effect of acupuncture is that in China it has been used in place of anaesthetics during operations.

Apart from the twelve meridians there are eight other intersecting channels through which the Ki energy flows. These are known as the strange flows of acupressure. Points are located along these paths which can be tapped by light touch to improve the flow of energy through the body. This has the indirect effect of enhancing the function of organs, obliterating pain and reducing stress. These points are known in acupressure as Jin Shin Do or Shen Taoist points, and they are mapped out on specific zones around the body. They can be activated by the light touch of a finger, and as they can be tender at times locating them should not be difficult. Once a zone is established the pressure can be applied for a few seconds before moving on to another point. It is worth mentioning also, at this stage, that tenderness on the skin surface can also be explained physiologically. Specific areas on the

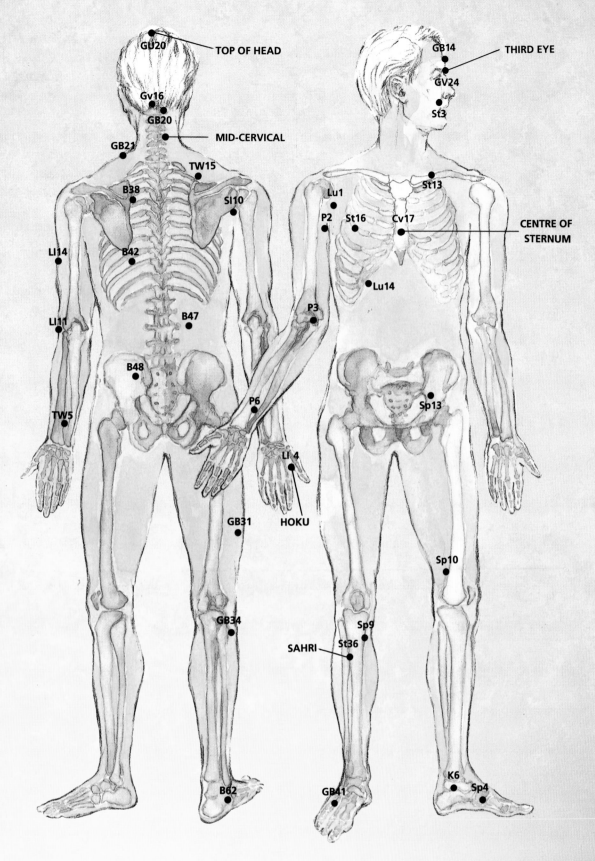

GV20 — TOP OF HEAD
Gv16
GB20 — MID-CERVICAL
GB21
TW15
B38
SI10
LI14
B42
LI11
B47
B48
TW5
P6
GB31 — HOKU
LI 4
GB34
B62

GB14 — THIRD EYE
GV24
St3
St13
Lu1
P2   St16   Cv17 — CENTRE OF STERNUM
Lu14
P3
Sp13
Sp10
Sp9
St36
SAHRI
K6   Sp4
GB41

The Acupressure points shown above are located in areas commonly used for acupuncture. They are, therefore, given acupuncture lettering and numbering, e.g Governing 16 (Gv16), Stomach 3 (St3), Spleen 10 (Sp10), Bladder 47 (B47) and so on. Most of the points are found bilaterally (i.e. on the right and left side of the body).

body surface relate to organs, glands, and joints, the connection being through nervous pathways between organs, spine, and skin. Any malfunction, inflammation, or disease will result in tenderness of one (or more) of these regions. Examples would be the presence of pain in the whole abdominal area in a case of appendicitis, and the pain in the shoulder relating to a liver or gall bladder problem. It is interesting to note that some of these reflex areas correlate to energy points.

I have found that treating these specific points with light touch has been very beneficial in some situations. I shall be using some of these points in this book, not as a treatment in itself, which would take a long time and is more suitable for a trained person, but as a beneficial addition to the massage techniques.

GIVING ACUPRESSURE MASSAGE

Although referred to as massage, there are no strokes and no sliding of the fingers or hands. The technique involves the appli-

cation of gentle light pressure with the fingers on **acupressure points** and holding this position for a few seconds.

In Chinese medicine the location of each point is very specific due to the precise location of the energy channel itself. Acupressure points are given letters and numbers which correspond to those mapped out in acupuncture. Most points are found in pairs, i.e. one on the left-hand side of the body and one on the right. Some are single points, usually in the mid-line of the body.

To receive an acupressure treatment the recipient lies down on their back or stomach. It is also possible, and in some cases preferred, to treat some points with the recipient sitting down. This is essential when carrying out a self treatment.

· ·

ACUPRESSURE MASSAGE

In some cases points are treated in pairs which implies applying pressure to the equivalent acupressure points on the left and right side of the body at the same time. At other times, two different points on the same side of the body are treated together. An example of two single points being treated with the recipient sitting down is shown here.

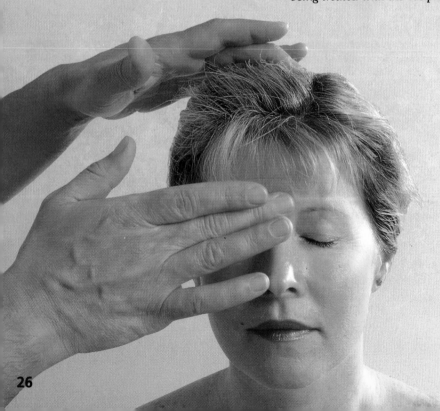

1 Stand on one side of the recipient. Place the middle finger of one hand on the **Top of head (GV20)** and the middle finger of the second hand on the **Third eye (GV24)** located between the eyebrows. Apply a little pressure to each point and hold this for a few seconds. Then gently ease the pressure and lift off your fingers.

REFLEXOLOGY

Reflexology is the term used for massage to specific areas of the feet. Called reflex points, they relate to the organs and to all other parts of the body. Massaging these points has a beneficial effect.

Reflexology originated as a result of the work of the American physician Dr William Fitzgerald. Having graduated in medicine at the University of Vermont in 1895, he travelled to Europe to work in a number of hospitals. In the early 1900s he developed the theory that a practitioner can have a considerable influence on the body organs by applying finger pressure to certain zones. His theory was based on the Chinese philosophy of treating the body with pressure or needles on specific points as in acupressure or acupuncture. Whereas the Chinese method was based on the twelve meridians through which

the energy is said to flow, Dr Fitzgerald discovered, or claimed, only ten areas which he called zones. It seems that his treatment also differed from the Chinese in that the pressure points were located mostly on the feet, and not throughout the whole body.

Dr Fitzgerald's method was taken up by Eunice D. Ingham, an American masseuse. While still maintaining that the treatment was based on the Chinese philosophy of energy pathways going through the organs of the body and the feet, Mrs Ingham talked about the pressure points on the feet as being areas

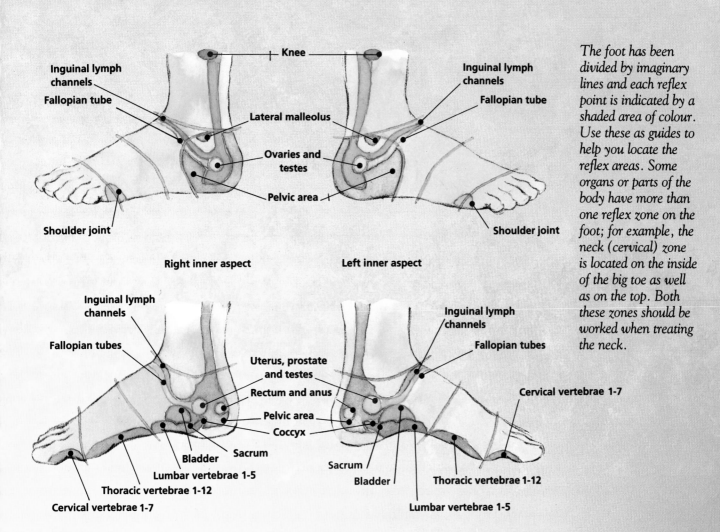

Left outer aspect **Right outer aspect**

Inguinal lymph channels
Fallopian tube
Knee
Lateral malleolus
Ovaries and testes
Pelvic area
Shoulder joint

Inguinal lymph channels
Fallopian tube
Shoulder joint

Right inner aspect **Left inner aspect**

Inguinal lymph channels
Fallopian tubes
Uterus, prostate and testes
Rectum and anus
Pelvic area
Coccyx
Bladder   Sacrum
Lumbar vertebrae 1-5
Thoracic vertebrae 1-12
Cervical vertebrae 1-7

Inguinal lymph channels
Fallopian tubes
Cervical vertebrae 1-7
Sacrum
Bladder
Thoracic vertebrae 1-12
Lumbar vertebrae 1-5

The foot has been divided by imaginary lines and each reflex point is indicated by a shaded area of colour. Use these as guides to help you locate the reflex areas. Some organs or parts of the body have more than one reflex zone on the foot; for example, the neck (cervical) zone is located on the inside of the big toe as well as on the top. Both these zones should be worked when treating the neck.

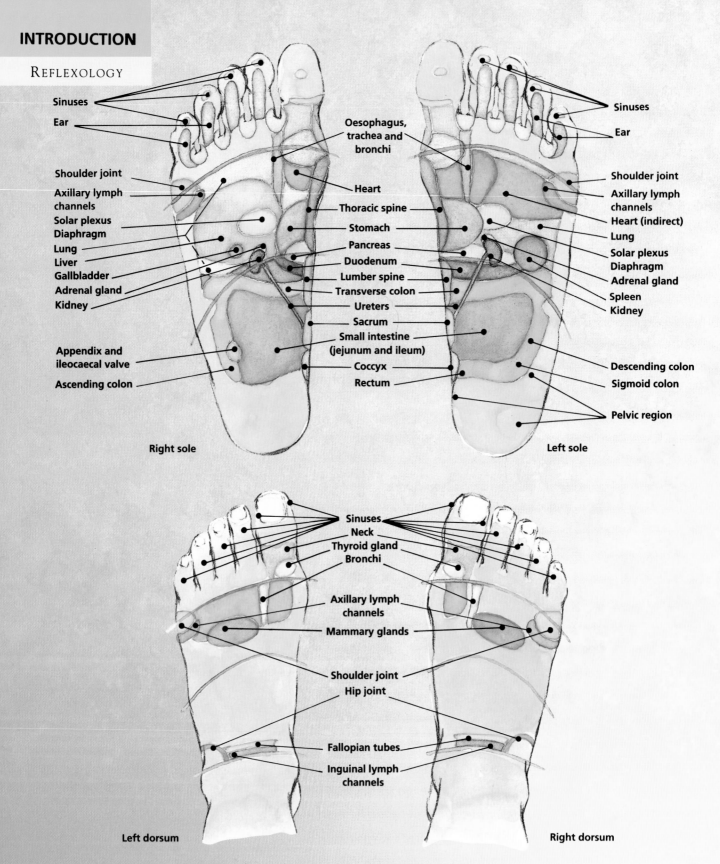

Sinuses
Ear
Shoulder joint
Axillary lymph channels
Solar plexus
Diaphragm
Lung
Liver
Gallbladder
Adrenal gland
Kidney

Appendix and ileocaecal valve

Ascending colon

Oesophagus, trachea and bronchi
Heart
Thoracic spine
Stomach
Pancreas
Duodenum
Lumber spine
Transverse colon
Ureters
Sacrum
Small intestine (jejunum and ileum)
Coccyx
Rectum

Sinuses
Ear
Shoulder joint
Axillary lymph channels
Heart (indirect)
Lung
Solar plexus
Diaphragm
Adrenal gland
Spleen
Kidney

Descending colon
Sigmoid colon

Pelvic region

Right sole

Left sole

Sinuses
Neck
Thyroid gland
Bronchi

Axillary lymph channels
Mammary glands

Shoulder joint
Hip joint

Fallopian tubes

Inguinal lymph channels

Left dorsum

Right dorsum

where tiny crystallizations can be found. Her explanation of these crystallizations, as expounded in her book *The Stories the Feet Can Tell (1938)*, was concerned with the nerve endings on the feet "reflexing" an organ, for example, the liver. She added that these crystal-like formations interfere with the circulation of the blood to the organ, preventing it from function-ing normally. Gentle thumb pressure is applied at the nerve endings to reduce the crystallization and so improve the function of the related organ. Whether we believe in the physiological explana-tion or the one based on the Chinese phi-losophy of energy, reflexology, or reflex zone therapy, as it is also called, has been found to benefit many areas and functions of the body and to help with the treatment of several ailments.

Some of the more common reflex points are shown in this book. As with the acupressure points, the use of these reflex points on the feet is not meant to constitute a full reflex zone therapy treatment. This can only be carried out by a trained therapist, but in my experience the reflex points included here can be used safely alongside massage.

REFLEX POINTS MASSAGE

Reflexology massage can be given with the recipient sitting on a chair or lying down. Cushions can be used to rest the foot being worked on and to raise it to a suitable height. No oil is required.

To locate a reflex point refer to the diagrams on pages 27–8. Massage the point by applying a gentle on-off pressure with the tip of your thumb. The recipient may experience a sharpish pain in the area if that particular point needs treating. You can still massage the zones if no pain is elicited but do not press too hard in an attempt to cause a reaction. To treat a point continue with the on–off thumb pressure on the same area for a few seconds or until the tenderness is reduced. Having worked on one point move on to another. Treatment can be repeated on any of the points during the same session. An example of a reflexology massage is given below.

REFLEX MASSAGE TO THE SOLAR PLEXUS

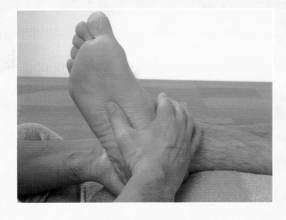

1 The recipient lies supine. Raise the foot on cushions and support it with both hands. Use the thumb to locate the reflex point.

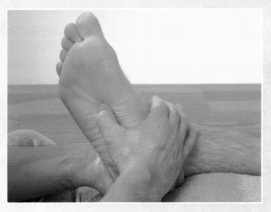

2 Apply the on-off pressure on the reflex zone. You may feel tiny crystallizations which should reduce as you massage. You need to be guided by the feedback from the recipient as to the extent and reduction of any discomfort.

The solar plexus is a major nerve junction situated in the abdomen just below the rib cage. It is also an anatomical point where tensions tend to be held. Massaging the reflex points on the feet which relate to the solar plexus can induce relaxation. It can be carried out at the beginning, or at the end of a relaxing massage routine.

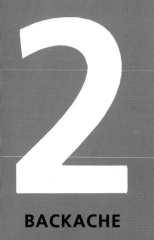
BACKACHE

"Lower back pain" is one of the commonest complaints encountered by doctors, and one of the most frequent reasons for absenteeism from work.

Approximately 30 per cent of the population is estimated to suffer from backache at any given time, and four out of five people will suffer from backache at some time during their life. Backache, in Britain alone, is estimated to cost £350,000,000 each year in medical costs and absenteeism.

The lower back is the area most susceptible to problems, pain here often being referred to as lumbago. This is a non-specific term and refers to discomfort ranging from an intermittent dull ache to a more acute sharp pain across the loin. The most common symptom is a vague sort of backache. It can result from sitting or standing for long periods, from driving, from doing housework, from decorating and gardening and from unfamiliar exercise. The discomfort arises from stiffness (spasm) of the muscles that are involved with maintaining posture and with bending and twisting.

The by-products of muscle work include carbon dioxide, lactic acid and water, all of which need to be cleared away by the circulation to avoid "clogging up" the muscle tissue. When the muscle is overworked or the circulation impaired, these products collect around the muscle and irritate the sensory nerve endings, producing a dull ache which varies in severity. Massage increases the circulation through the muscle tissue, helping to remove the waste products and consequently reducing stiffness and pain.

A build-up of fluid in the area of the lower back, causing pressure, can also be a cause of backache. This can happen after an injury, like a back strain. It can also be associated with hormonal changes like those of menstruation, and with arthritic conditions. Lymph drainage techniques can be used to assist the movement of the fluid.

Backache can be complicated in some people by an increased lumbar curvature, known medically as lordosis, where the back is extremely hollow. This can lead to a number of problems including compression of the lumbar spine, disc damage, arthritis and fluid retention. Such conditions require the attention of a general practitioner or a complementary therapist specialising in body mechanics.

PRECAUTIONS

An accurate diagnosis of the cause of low back pain is one of the most difficult a doctor has to make. While it is usually caused by minor strains or injuries this is not always the case. For example, kidney problems can lead to vague back pain which varies in severity. Slipped discs produce very severe acute pain with most movements. Muscle strains are very common and these, too, produce an acute sharp pain that intensifies with movement. Both slipped discs and muscle strains may result from postural problems or injury. They are likely to lead to inflammation of a main nerve root and to the accompanying pain of sciatica, which radiates down the back of the leg. Misalignments of the spine are not necessarily as incapacitating, and the pain is more likely to be a persistent ache that can become sharp upon movement. Any of these conditions can be experienced after heavy lifting, taking part in sports, making sudden movements or doing unaccustomed physical work. As well as the local area of discomfort there can be radiating pain, loss of sensation, loss of muscle strength, a sensation of heat or cold or that of pins and needles. Affected areas may include the loin, the abdomen, the pelvis and the legs and feet.

Problems like these are best treated

EXERCISES FOR THE LOWER BACK

1 Lie on your back on the floor. Hold your knees with both hands and bring them towards your chest. Do not cause any unnecessary pain by pulling too much. Breathe in deeply, and as you breathe out gently pull your knees further towards your chest. Repeat several times.

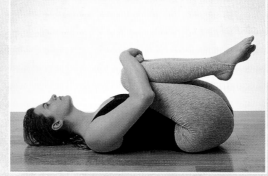

These exercises can be used to ease muscle stiffness and are useful in cases of increased lumbar curvature. They should not be done if any form of muscle strain exists.

2 Stand facing a heavy table, banister, kitchen worktop or something similar which is not likely to move. Stand about 45 cm (18 in) away and grip the table with both hands. Bend forward from the hips keeping your knees locked straight at the same time. Your back should now be in a straight horizontal line. Push your buttocks backwards to stretch the lower back. Hold the position for a few breaths, increasing the stretch on breathing out.

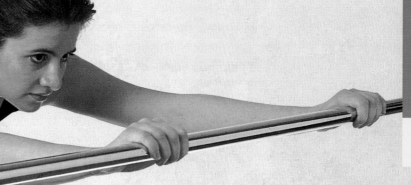

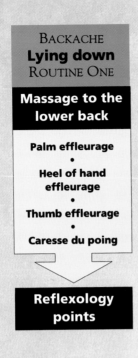

BACKACHE
Lying down
ROUTINE ONE

Massage to the lower back

Palm effleurage
•
Heel of hand effleurage
•
Thumb effleurage
•
Caresse du poing

Reflexology points

BACKACHE
Lying down
ROUTINE TWO

Massage to the upper back and shoulders

Palm effleurage
•
Criss-cross effleurage
•
Reinforced palm effleurage
•
Thumb effleurage
•
Caresse du poing

Take care not to:
....
**Massage the lower back if there is:
Unexplained heat or inflammation
•
Build-up of fluid associated with conditions such as cancer or heart problems
•
Severe pain on movement or on palpitating the area with the fingers**

by a general practitioner or a manipulative therapist such as an osteopath. Massage, therefore, is not likely to be used in such situations and if it is, only by a qualified massage therapist.

SELF-HELP SUGGESTIONS

The following are pointers to help you recognize the symptoms associated with lower back problems, and advice on how to deal with the situation until proper treatment is available.

Acute, sharp pain: Very acute, sharp pain which increases considerably on any movement no matter how small. This kind of pain is very severe on turning over in bed, on sitting up or down, and on bending forward even slightly. There may be accompanying pain or sensations elsewhere. Apply a cold wet towel to the lower back. This helps to reduce fluid build-up and inflammation. A small folded towel is dipped in cold water (straight from the tap) and any excess wrung out. It is then applied to the area for about ten minutes. The towel is turned over and refreshed in the cold water frequently to keep the tissues cool. Lie down in whichever is the most comfortable position and rest until the pain subsides sufficiently to move about or until you can get medical help.

Heat: Considerable heat in the lower back area but with movement not very restricted could suggest some nerve root inflammation. In this situation apply a cold wet towel in the morning and last thing at night and seek advice as early as possible.

Dull ache: A dull ache associated with sitting for long periods or doing physical work like gardening or decorating could be caused by muscle stiffness. Apply heat in the form of hot towels, a hot bath, or a hot-water bottle. Consult your doctor or a manipulative therapist if the pain does not subside or if it recurs over the following few days after the activity has stopped.

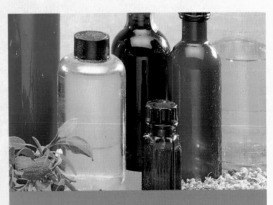

ESSENTIAL OILS
....

Use for aching, tight and stiff muscles. These oils have a very analgesic effect.

**Rosemary • Marjoram
• Camomile • Lavender**

Use one essence or a mixture of two and put about five drops in a hot bath. They can also be mixed with a carrier oil and used for massage. Use 2% essence to carrier oil.

THE LOWER BACK

The following routine is used for lower back ache. The time required for the routine can be varied to suit the recipient, but 20 minutes is an average.

PALM EFFLEURAGE

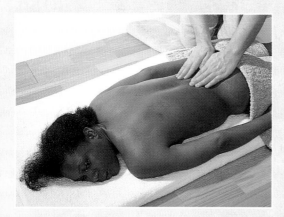

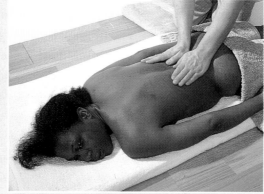

1 Start at the upper end of the buttocks. Place your hands beside the spine, one on each side, with the whole hand contacting the skin and the fingers pointing towards the head. Effleurage with both hands at the same time towards the head.

2 Keep your hands very close to the spine and make contact with the whole palm. Effleurage upwards until your hands reach the lower rib cage, then rotate the fingers towards the outside of the trunk.

This effleurage increases the circulation to the area and relaxes the recipient, as well as beginning to relax the muscles. Repeat the movement several times or until the recipient feels it is time to stop. A cushion can be placed underneath the abdomen for added comfort.

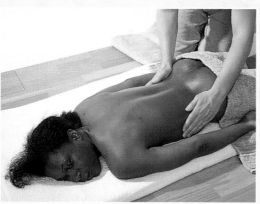

3 With your hands still in this position effleurage down towards the buttocks. Reduce the pressure as you carry out this stroke. When the hands reach the buttocks move them towards each other to meet in the centre, then rotate the fingers to point towards the head and repeat the movement.

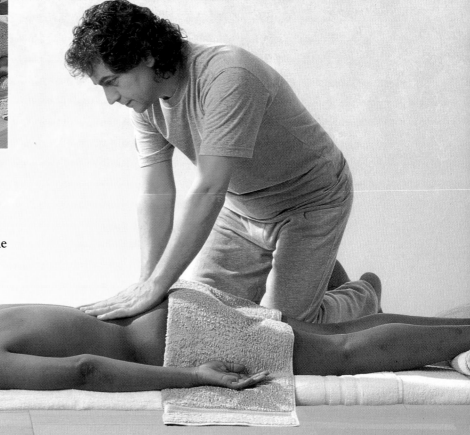

This movement is a palm effleurage but with the emphasis on the heel of the hand. It is used to relax the muscle tissue and to stretch it sideways, towards the side of the trunk. Apply this technique after the area has been warmed up with the palm effleurage described previously. Do not use this stroke over the kidney area. Repeat the movement several times or until the recipient feels it is time to stop.

HEEL OF HAND EFFLEURAGE

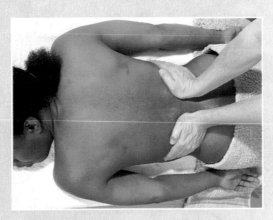
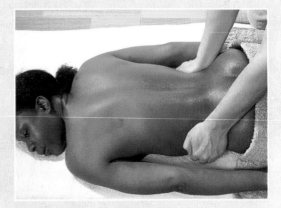

1 Start the stroke by placing both hands very close to the spine with the fingers pointing towards the outside of the trunk. The hands follow the curve of the trunk and contact is made with the whole palm and fingers.

2 Apply pressure with the heel of the hand as you effleurage outwards. Ease off the pressure as your fingertips touch the surface on which the recipient is lying, and as the heel of the hand passes over the softer tissues. Return to the starting position and repeat.

REPEAT TECHNIQUES

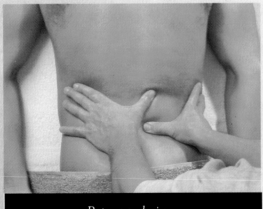

Repeat technique
· · · · · · · · · · · · · · · · · · · ·
THUMB EFFLEURAGE
See page 19
·
Follows HEEL OF HAND EFFLEURAGE

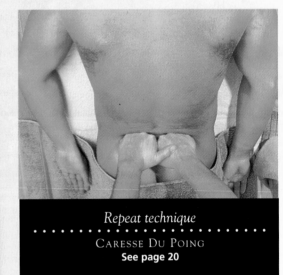

Repeat technique
· · · · · · · · · · · · · · · · · · · ·
CARESSE DU POING
See page 20
·
Follows THUMB EFFLEURAGE

REFLEX POINTS –
SPINE AND LOWER BACK

1 Support the foot either on a cushion or on
your lap. Use one hand to hold the foot
while the second hand applies the pressure
with the thumb. The area to be reflexed is on
the instep just below the bones. You may need
to find the exact points by feeling for them
with your thumb. When you touch a reflex
point which needs treating the recipient will
report a sharpish pain, or the tissues under
your thumb may feel "gritty".

Once a point has been located, treat the
area by applying an on-off pressure as the
thumb compresses for a second before it is
eased off again. Continue with this technique
for six to ten seconds before moving to
another point.

Treatment of all the reflex points located
can be repeated in the same session if
necessary.

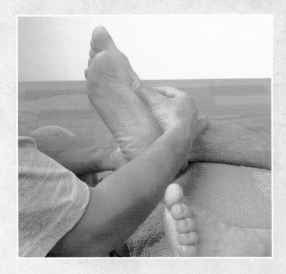

*The area on the foot
which reflects the
lumbar spine is on the
instep. There are
some prominent
bones here and the
thumb should, more
or less, follow these.*

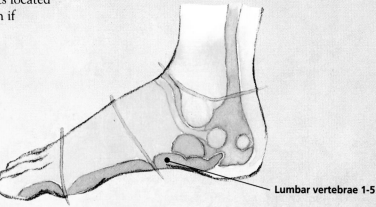

Lumbar vertebrae 1-5

SELF-ADMINISTERED
REFLEX POINT MASSAGE

1 Locate the point or points as indicated
earlier, that is by feeling with the thumb
for any tender areas. Treat a point by applying
on-off thumb pressure for about six to ten
seconds. Move on to another reflex point.
When you have treated all the points which
are tender return to the first one and repeat
the process.

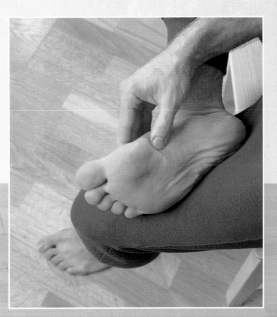

*To treat the reflex
points yourself, sit on
a chair or on the floor
and place one foot on
the opposite thigh.*

UPPER BACK AND SHOULDERS

The upper back and shoulders are very susceptible to pain related to posture and work. In some people the spine in the upper back develops a forward-bending curve that may be the result of an habitual posture or the shape the bones take during growing up. Muscles in this area are likely to tense to counterbalance this posture. Massage is used to reduce this tension.

PALM EFFLEURAGE

This effleurage is used to increase the circulation, to warm up the area and for relaxation. It can be repeated several times.

Take care not to:

Massage if any of the following symptoms are present:
Severe pain on pressing the back with the fingers

•

Unexplained excessive heat

•

Pain which radiates to the arms or the rib cage

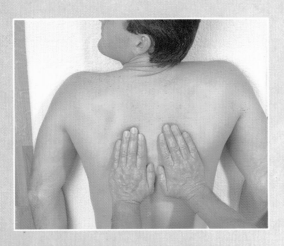

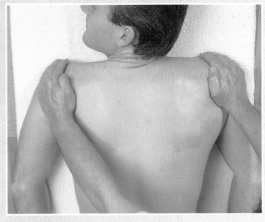

1 Place the hands on each side of the spine with the fingers pointing towards the head. Be careful to avoid pressing on the spine itself. Starting at the middle of the back effleurage upwards towards the head.

2 Continue the movement outwards to include the shoulders. Cup your hands as you effleurage round the shoulders.

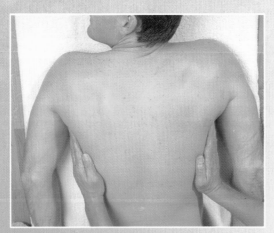

3 Then ease off the pressure, maintain contact with your palm and fingers and effleurage the outside of the trunk moving your hands towards the feet. Turn the heel of each hand towards the spine and move the hands to meet in the middle of the back. Turn the fingers so that they are pointing towards the head again and repeat the movement.

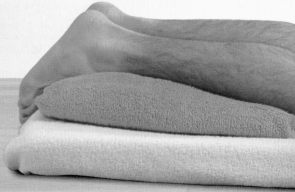

CRISS-CROSS EFFLEURAGE

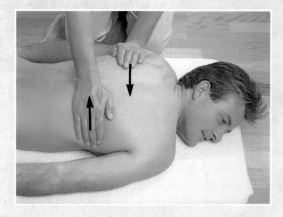

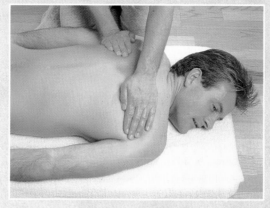

Criss-cross effleurage can be used in addition to palm effleurage for general relaxation and warming up.

1 Place one hand beside the spine on the side nearest to you and the other hand on the opposite side, with the fingers of both hands pointing away from you.

2 Make contact with the palms and fingers and effleurage by moving the hands in opposite directions across the back.

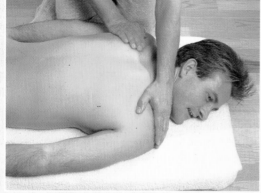

4 Carry on with the criss-cross effleurage stroke working downwards to the middle of the back again. This movement is carried out very slowly and repeated several times for a relaxing effect.

3 Start at the middle of the back and continue the movement upwards to include the shoulders and upper arms.

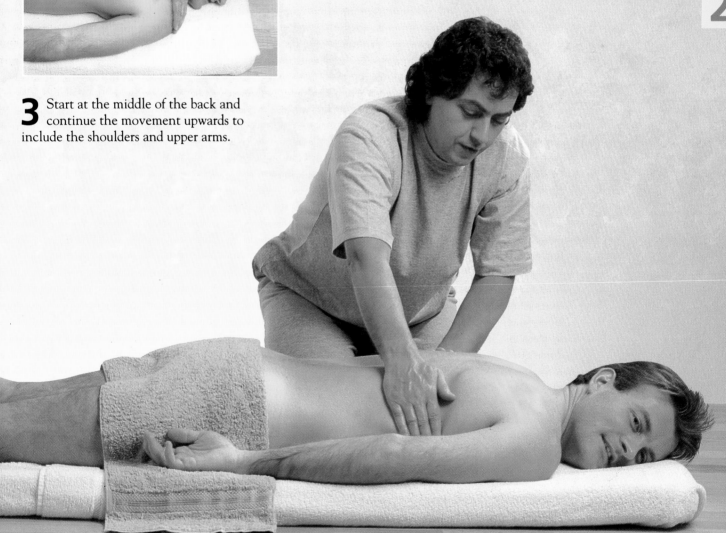

REINFORCED PALM EFFLEURAGE – SHOULDERS

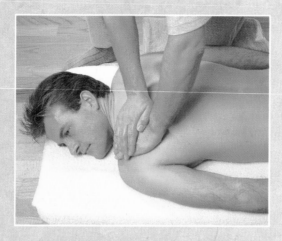

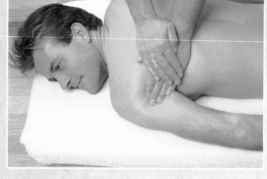

Reinforced palm effleurage allows you to increase the pressure when massaging heavy muscular areas like the shoulders.

1 Reach over to the opposite shoulder. Use one hand reinforced by the other to cup and effleurage round the shoulder.

2 Start at the top end of the shoulder and continue the movement round towards the outside.

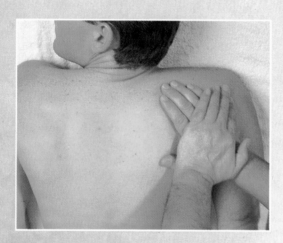

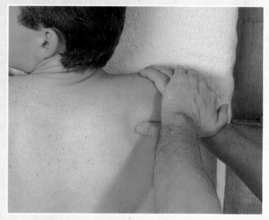

3 The same movement can be carried out on the shoulder nearest to you. Place your hands in the same position as for the other side, one hand on top of the other with pressure being applied mostly by the top hand.

4 Starting from the upper part of the shoulder, effleurage round to the outside and over the upper arm area.

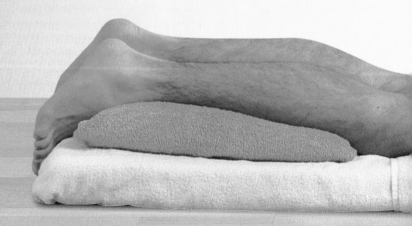

THUMB EFFLEURAGE – SCAPULA

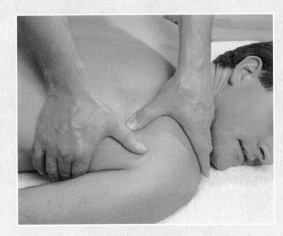

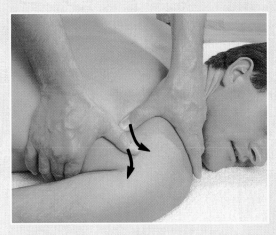

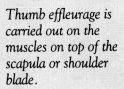

Thumb effleurage is carried out on the muscles on top of the scapula or shoulder blade.

1 Position yourself on one side of the recipient and place both hands on the shoulder blade on the opposite side.

2 Use the same thumb position as for the rhomboids (see page 40). Keeping the hands in this position, effleurage to cover as much of the shoulder blade area as possible.

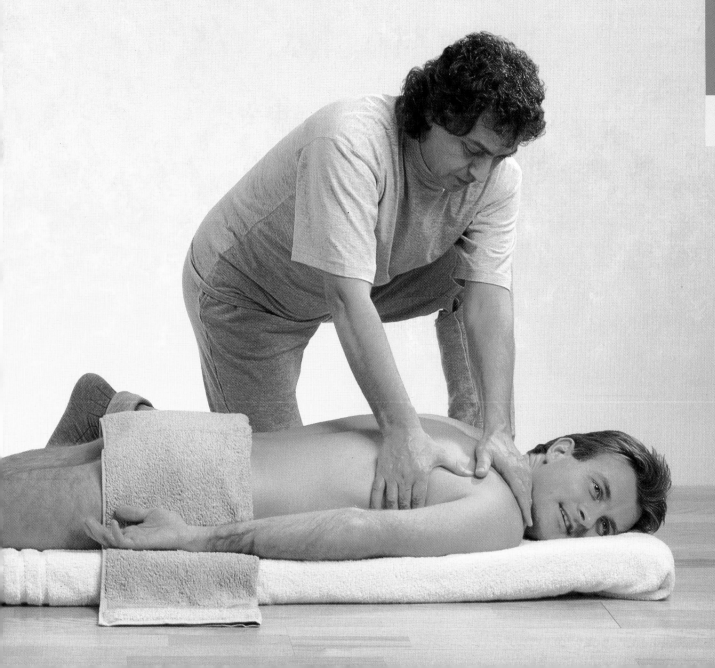

THUMB EFFLEURAGE – UPPER BACK
(RHOMBOIDS AREA)

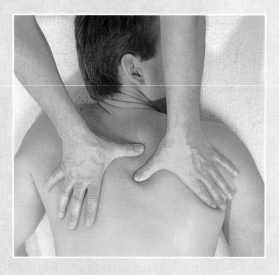

The rhomboid muscles run across from the spine to the shoulder blade, and are frequently tense. These muscles are massaged with the thumbs (digital effleurage).

1 Position yourself at the head of the recipient. Place both hands on the upper back with the thumbs to one side of the spine.

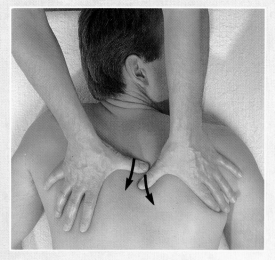

2 The stroke is done with the thumb, pressing into the muscles in the direction of the feet for about 5cm (2 in).

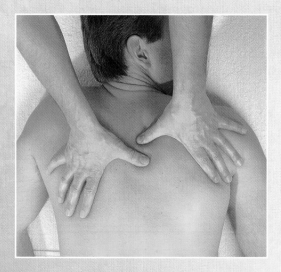

3 Carry out the movement alternately with each thumb. Each stroke of the thumb can also involve the hand moving in the same direction but not applying as much pressure.

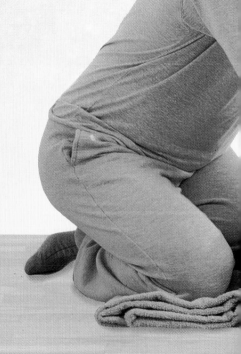

CARESSE DU POING

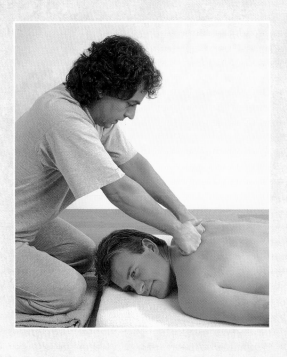

1 Position yourself at the head of the recipient. Place the back of each hand, closed in a fist, one on each side of the spine. Effleurage in the direction of the lower back with each fist, making sure that only the flat part of the fist is used and not the knuckles.

If extra pressure is required for tense muscles in this area, the caresse du poing technique is especially suitable.

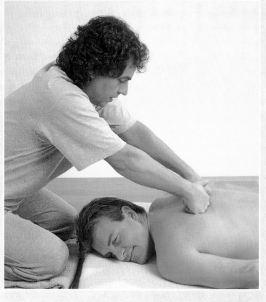

2 Continue the stroke until you reach the middle of the back, or to wherever feels a comfortable point to stop. Lift the hands off and return to the first position to repeat the stroke.

3

TENSION HEADACHE

. . . .

A headache may be described in ways which reflect either its location or its severity, for example it may occur over the forehead, over the eyes, or across the top of the head, and we may call it a splitting headache, a throbbing pain or an intermittent ache.

Tension headache, as the term implies, is due to tension or stress. The kinds of tension that can contribute to a headache are twofold: constriction in artery walls, leading to a raising of the blood pressure to the head; excessive tension in neck and shoulder muscles. The increased blood pressure is transmitted to the cerebrospinal fluid (a fluid which flows through the central nervous system) just below the skull and makes the head feel as if it is about to burst. Muscle tightness affects the spine and in turn the spinal nerves. Some of these supply the scalp and, when irritated, can cause pain across the top of the head to the forehead.

Stress can be greatly reduced not only by dealing with its causes but also by massage techniques and relaxation methods like visualization. A number of massage oils are recommended for their anti-stress properties (see left). This approach can be supplemented with massage work on acupressure points and reflex zones.

The upper part of the back and lower neck are often found to be misaligned when tension headache is present. This implies a small degree of misplacement and the locking of two adjoining vertebrae (spinal bones) and happens as a result of postural problems or injury. It can result in the spinal nerves, which emerge from between the vertebrae, being irritated or inflamed. This can lead to a neuralgia-type pain radiating to the top of the head, or a sensation of pins and needles along the arms and hands.

The muscles of the upper shoulders and neck are very much involved in this kind of problem. Stiffness of this muscle group can result in the spine locking, and spinal misalignment will result in these muscles tensing up and being painful. Massage is used to help break this vicious circle by relaxing the muscles. In some cases, however, the most effective treatment for spinal misalignments is manipu-

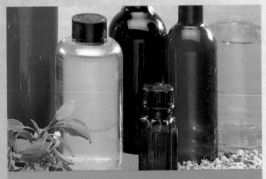

MASSAGE OILS FOR RELAXATION

. . . .

Oils to help relax muscles
**Marjoram • Lavender
• Camomile • Rosemary**

Oils to help reduce tension
**Bergamot • Camomile
• Clary sage • Jasmine • Lavender
• Marjoram • Neroli • Rose**

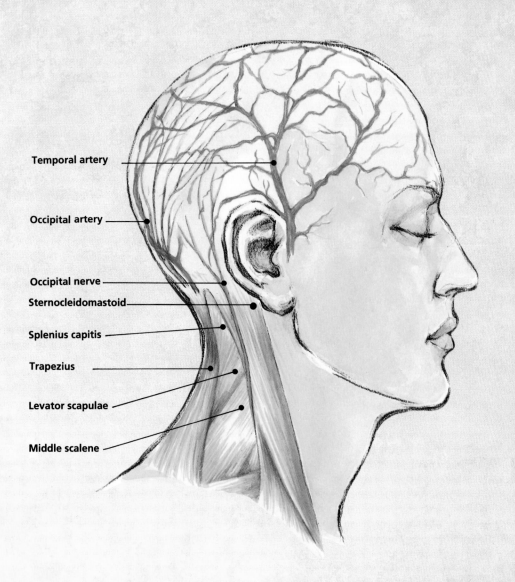

Temporal artery

Occipital artery

Occipital nerve

Sternocleidomastoid

Splenius capitis

Trapezius

Levator scapulae

Middle scalene

Nerves travel from the upper neck area to the back and top of the head, supplying the skin and underlying muscles. Blood vessels also supply the same tissues and therefore are widespread throughout the head. Tightness of the neck muscles can affect the nerves and blood vessels, resulting in tension headache.

lation by an osteopath or chiropractor. Nonetheless, massage can help reduce the stiffness and pain in the muscles.

PRECAUTIONS

Headaches can be precipitated by illness like infections and viruses, and by the intake of narcotics. Massage should not be given in such circumstances and medical advice should be sought. For example: alcohol excess; smoking; chills; medicinal drugs like quinine, morphine, atropine and histamine; infections such as those of the throat, ear, sinuses and gall bladder; fevers; meningitis.

TENSION HEADACHE **Sitting** ROUTINE ONE	TENSION HEADACHE **Lying down** ROUTINE TWO	TENSION HEADACHE **Self-administered**
Palm effleurage • Thumb effleurage • Kneading • Pick-up effleurage • Scalp massage	Palm effleurage • Thumb effleurage – upper back • Kneading • Pick-up effleurage • Thumb effleurage – head	Kneading • Digital effleurage – head • Scalp massage
		Acupressure
Acupressure	**Acupressure**	
Reflexology		

43

TENSION HEADACHE: SITTING

You can use the following sequence, or a selection of techniques. The routine starts with palm effleurage and finishes with reflex points on the feet. Allow between 20 and 30 minutes. The recipient sits on a chair.

PALM EFFLEURAGE – NECK AND SHOULDERS

The muscles of the neck and shoulders can hold a great amount of tension. A muscle which is not ready to relax will tense up even more if heavy massage is carried out. Relaxation of these muscles, therefore, must not be rushed. Palm effleurage is used to start the process and may need to be done for quite a while before deeper massage techniques are used.

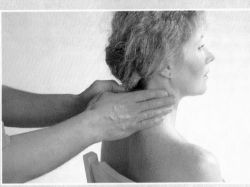

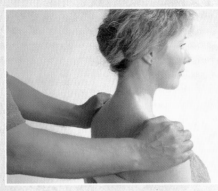

1 Sit the recipient in a chair, preferably one with a low back, and stand behind it. Place your hands on either side of the neck.

2 Making contact mostly with the palm of the hand, start at the top and effleurage down the neck. Continue the movement to the shoulders.

3 As you go over the top of the shoulders use the fingers as well as the palm of the hand to increase the pressure slightly. When you reach the outside of the shoulders return the hands to the top of the neck without losing contact with the skin. Repeat several times maintaining a slow rhythm.

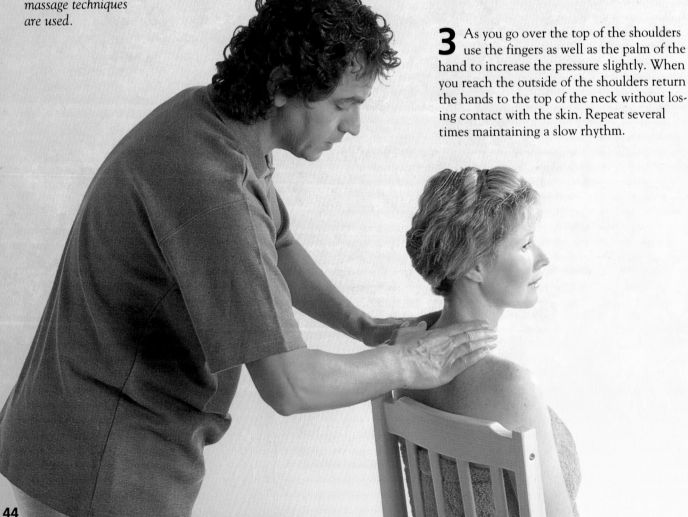

THUMB EFFLEURAGE –
UPPER BACK AND TOP OF SHOULDERS

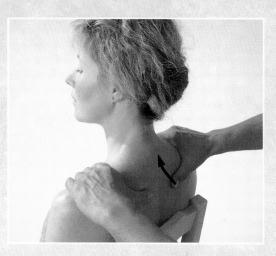

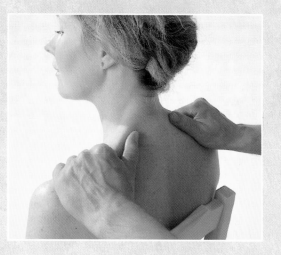

To work more deeply into the muscles thumb effleurage is applied. The pressure is adjusted according to the "give" in the muscles – as you feel them relaxing it is gradually increased.

1 Place one hand on each shoulder. The fingers should be over the shoulder and the thumb between the spine and the shoulder blade. Gently apply pressure with the thumb of each hand as you move it towards the top of the shoulder.

2 The fingers and palm can apply a gentle squeeze while the thumb is applying most of the pressure. The thumb is lifted as it gets near to the fingers, so as not to pinch the skin. Repeat the movement several times increasing the pressure with each stroke.

KNEADING – UPPER BACK AND SHOULDERS

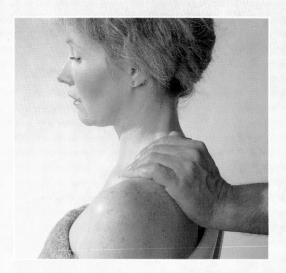

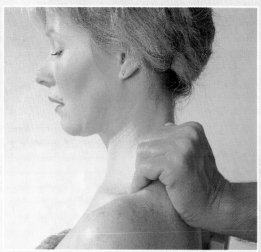

The kneading in this technique refers to a gentle squeeze between the heel of the hand and the fingertips. The main muscle which benefits from this movement is the upper part of the trapezius, which runs from the neck to the outside of the shoulder. The effect of the stroke is to encourage the circulation through the muscle and at the same time to stretch it slightly across its length. The movement is best carried out on one shoulder at a time.

1 Stand slightly behind and to the side of the recipient. Place one hand on top of the opposite shoulder, in between the base of the neck and the outside of the shoulder. Gently lift and squeeze the muscle between the fingertips and the heel of the hand.

2 Continue the squeeze but let the heel of the hand move towards the fingertips so as to stretch the muscle across its fibres. Care must be taken not to pinch the skin as you come to the end of the stroke. Repeat several times.

Pick-up effleurage is used to relax and stretch the muscles at the back of the neck.

PICK-UP EFFLEURAGE – NECK

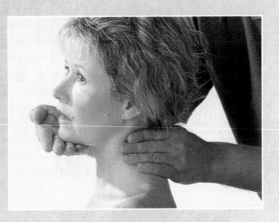

1 Stand to the side of the recipient. Support the chin with one hand. Place the other hand at the back of the neck with your fingers on one side and your thumb on the other side. Compress the neck muscles gently between the fingers and the thumb.

2 Continue with the compression as you begin to stretch the muscles and overlying skin away from the spine. Ease off the pressure as the hand begins to slide off to ensure that the skin is not being pinched.

THUMB EFFLEURAGE–BACK OF THE HEAD

The bone running across the back of the head from ear to ear is called the occiput and it articulates with the first vertebra of the neck. It also acts as a place of attachment for the muscles at the back of the neck and the top of the shoulders. In this area of attachment there are several "trigger points", which can be described as the relay stations of nerve impulses. They are involved with muscle tension and in some instances with pain in the head. Working along the base of the occiput will help to relax muscles. This area can be very tender and therefore the pressure may need to be very light.

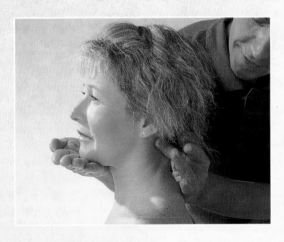

1 Stand at the side of the recipient. Support the chin with one hand, place the other hand at the back of the neck with the thumb underneath the occiput, just behind the ear. The middle finger is placed underneath the occiput behind the opposite ear. The stroke is being carried out with the right hand.

2 Apply equal pressure with the thumb and middle finger as you run them along the base of the occiput toward the center of the neck. When they meet at the center, lift them off and return to the starting position to repeat the movement. The stroke is being carried out with the left hand.

SCALP MASSAGE

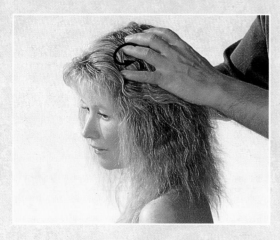

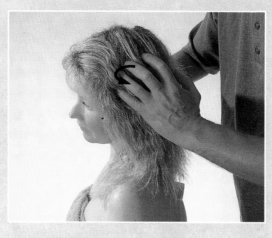

Scalp massage is one of the most relaxing forms of massage. It entails applying pressure with the fingertips to move the scalp over the skull. The movement leads to an increase in the local circulation and also to a great sense of relaxation. There is no need to use any oil for this movement.

1 Stand behind the recipient and place both hands on top of the head. Apply sufficient pressure with the fingertips (try not to use the thumbs) to move the scalp over the skull in small circles. If there is no movement or not much movement increase the pressure slightly. Some people's scalps are not easy to move, in which case the massage stroke is still applied but without any forceful pressure.

2 Having completed a few circles in the first position move the hands to a new position and repeat the stroke until eventually you cover most of the top and sides of the head.

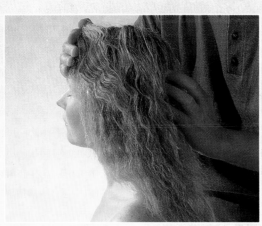

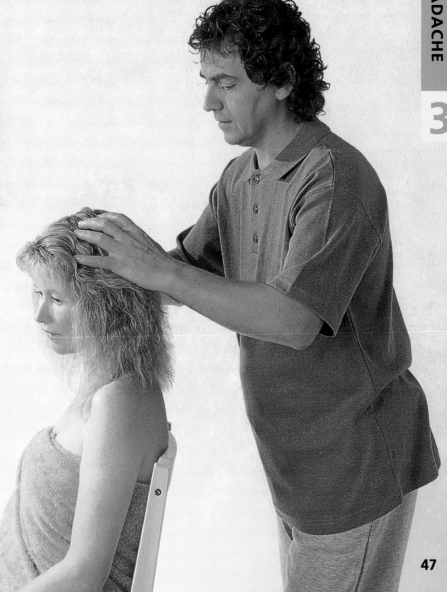

3 Stand at the side of the recipient so that you can now massage the back of the head. One hand is used for massaging while the other supports the forehead or chin. Massage in small circles again and move the hand position so as to cover the whole area at the back of the head.

ACUPRESSURE FOR RELAXATION

The illustrations show the location of the points. You may need to locate a point with your finger or thumb by feeling for any tender zones. Once located, the point can be treated with very light pressure for a few seconds. Some points are more tender than others, but whether tender or not they still should be treated. Usually points on the left and right sides of the body are worked on simultaneously. The recipient can be sitting or lying down depending on the points being treated. Use the following points as part of the massage routine to induce relaxation.

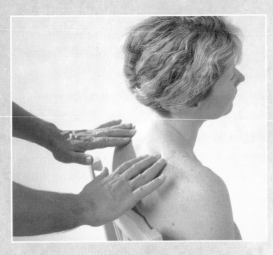

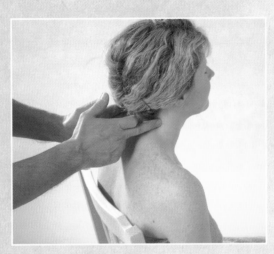

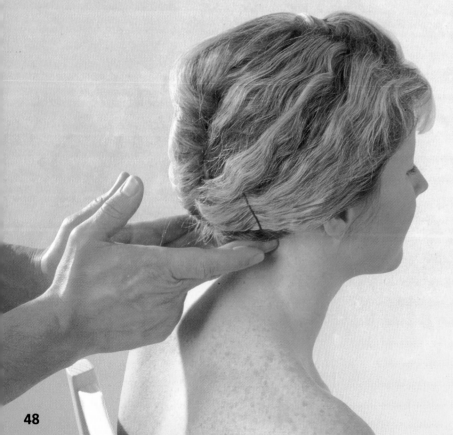

Point TW15: On either side of body. Treated simultaneously. **Location:** Slightly above the top corner of the shoulder blade nearest to the spine.

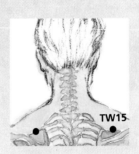

Point Mid-cervical: On either side of body. Treat simultaneously. **Location:** Halfway between the base of the skull and the lower end of the neck. To the side of the bony prominence. This point tends to be contra-indicated during pregnancy.

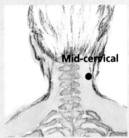

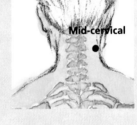

Point GB20: On either side of body. Treat simultaneously. **Location:** At the base of the skull. On each side of the spine, halfway between the spine and the bony prominence behind the ears, there is a tiny hollow in between two groups of muscles where this point is located.

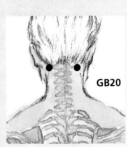

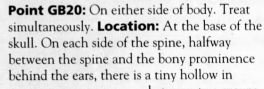

Point Top of head and **Point Third eye:** Treat simultaneously.
Location: Top of head (GV20) At the very centre of the top of the head. **Third eye** (GV24) The middle of the forehead between the eyebrows.

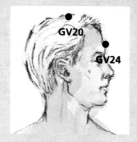

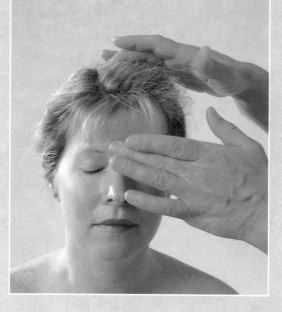

· ·

REFLEX POINTS – NECK

1 The reflex points for the neck are found at the base of the big toe, both on the inner surface and the top part of the toe.

2 Hold the foot with both hands. Use the thumb nearest to the big toe to locate and massage the inner reflex point. Once located apply intermittent pressure for a few seconds. This is done into the tissue and not in circles.

3 Repeat the movement on the reflex point situated on the top part of the toe. Then repeat both reflex points on the other foot.

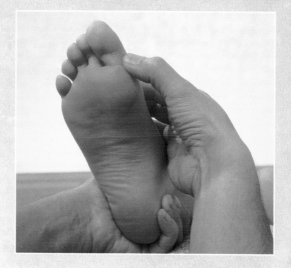

The reflex points on the feet can be massaged with the recipient lying supine, or sitting on a chair (with you sitting on a chair or stool opposite). The foot being massaged can rest on a cushion or towel placed on your lap. No oil is necessary for reflex point massage.

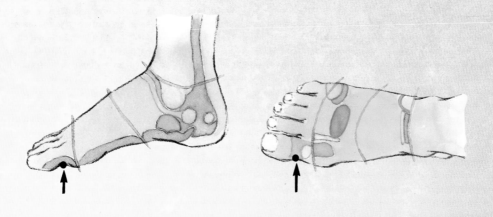

TENSION HEADACHE:LYING

The recipient lies face down for the following techniques. Techniques are like tools, they can be adapted to fit a number of applications. For example, a massage movement like effleurage can be applied with varying pressures and rhythms for different results. Movements are therefore carried out on the same area but for a different effect. The routine starts with palm effleurage and ends with acupressure points. Do not rush the sequence, which should take about 20 minutes.

THUMB EFFLEURAGE–UPPER BACK AND TOP OF SHOULDERS

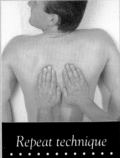

Repeat technique

PALM EFFLEURAGE –
UPPER BACK AND
TOP OF SHOULDERS
See page 36
•
Before
THUMB EFFLEURAGE
– UPPER BACK AND
SHOULDERS

To work more deeply into the muscles, thumb effleurage is used. Pressure is applied with the thumbs and adjusted according to the "give" of the muscles; that is, it is gradually increased as you feel the muscles relaxing with each stroke.

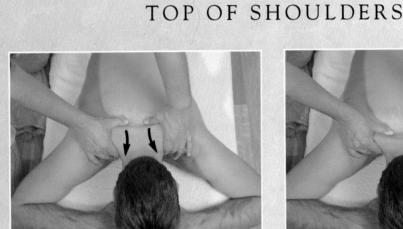

1 This technique follows Palm Effleurage. Kneel with one leg on either side of the recipient. Place one hand on each shoulder. The fingers of each hand are placed over the shoulder with the thumb in between the spine and the scapula (shoulder blade).

2 Gently apply pressure with the thumb of each hand as you move it towards the top of the shoulder. The fingers and palm can apply a gentle squeeze while the thumb applies most of the pressure.

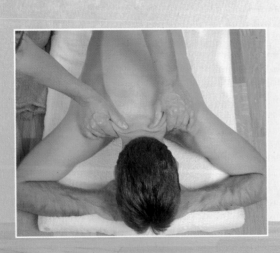

3 Lift the thumb as it nears the fingers, so as not to pinch the skin. Repeat the movement several times, aiming to increase the pressure with each stroke.

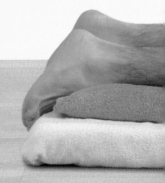

KNEADING –
UPPER BACK AND SHOULDERS

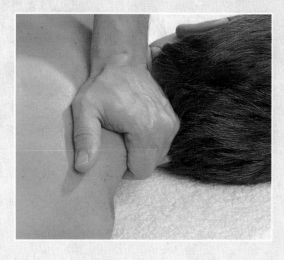

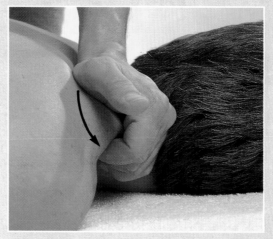

Single-handed petrissage is used to reduce muscle spasm. It is best to use the right hand on the right shoulder and the left hand on the left shoulder.

1 Position yourself to one side of the recipient. Turn the head towards you or let the forehead rest on the hands. Place one hand on the opposite shoulder. Gently lift the muscle while holding it between the fingers and the heel of the hand.

2 The heel of the hand applies some pressure as it moves towards the fingertips to squeeze and stretch the muscle across its fibres. The fingers act as a support for the muscle, and therefore apply very little pressure.

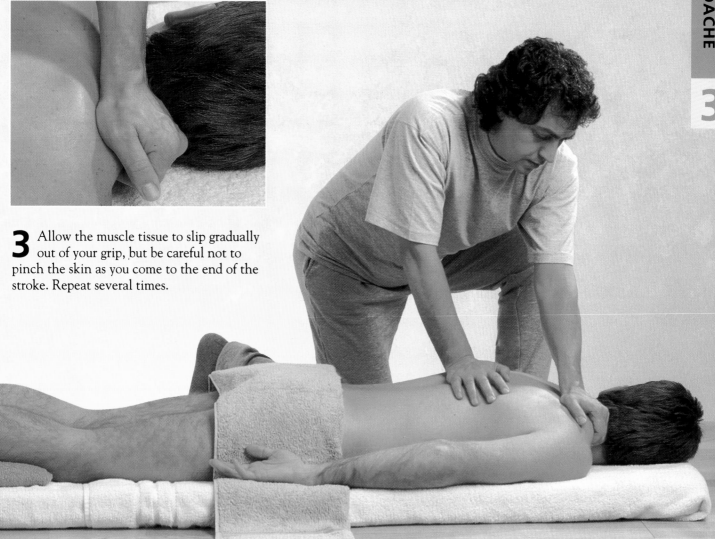

3 Allow the muscle tissue to slip gradually out of your grip, but be careful not to pinch the skin as you come to the end of the stroke. Repeat several times.

PICK-UP EFFLEURAGE – NECK MUSCLES

Pick-up effleurage gently compresses the muscles and tissues at the back of the neck and stretches them away from the spine. It can be repeated several times but the pressure does not increase with each stroke.

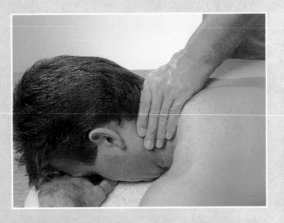

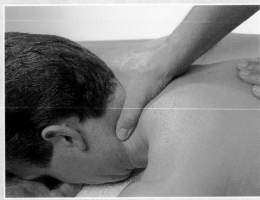

1 Position yourself to one side of the recipient. His or her head should rest on his or her hands which are placed on top of each other. Use one hand to compress the neck muscles gently between the fingers and the thumb.

2 Continue the compression as you begin to stretch the muscles and overlying tissues away from the spine. This picture demonstrates the thumb position (but with the left hand, rather than the right).

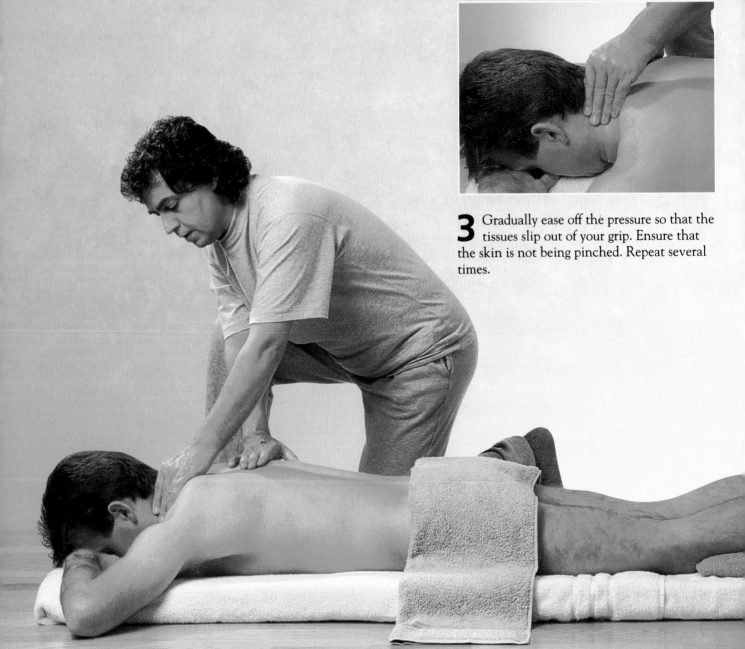

3 Gradually ease off the pressure so that the tissues slip out of your grip. Ensure that the skin is not being pinched. Repeat several times.

THUMB EFFLEURAGE–
BACK OF THE HEAD

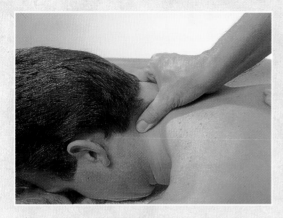

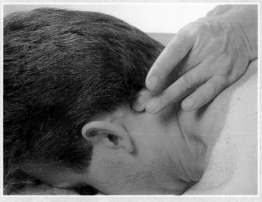

This movement has been described on page 46. The position of the massaging hand is still the same when the recipient is lying face down. Your second hand rests on the shoulder.

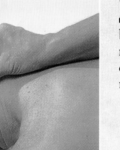

1 Position yourself to one side of the recipient. Place your thumb underneath the occipital bone, just behind the ear nearest to you. Your middle finger is placed behind the opposite ear.

2 Apply equal pressure with the thumb and middle finger as you run them along the base of the occiput towards the centre of the neck. When they meet at the centre, lift them off and return to the starting position to repeat the movement.

This movement has been described on page 46.

TENSION HEADACHE

3

ACUPRESSURE POINTS

1 Point Bladder 42: Located on the back, at the lower part of the rib cage. Imagine a line between the shoulder blade and the spine, but at a distance of two fingers' width below the lower end of the shoulder blade. The point is located at the halfway along this line.

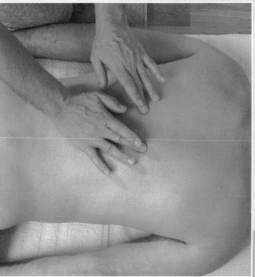

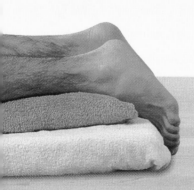

Position yourself to the side of the recipient to treat these points as a pair, one on each side of the body.

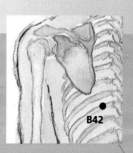

B42

TENSION HEADACHE: SELF-ADMINISTERED

Use these techniques in any sequence as a self-treatment to reduce tension headaches or for general relaxation, ideally after or during a hot bath.

KNEADING – UPPER BACK AND SHOULDERS

This technique works on the knotted muscles, which are associated with tension. Like all other techniques it is done in a leisurely manner.

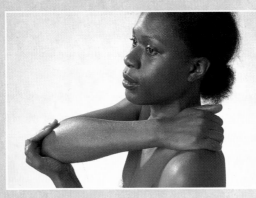
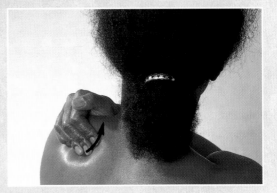

1 Sit on a chair or stool. Use one hand to massage the muscles of the opposite shoulder, and the second hand to support the elbow of the massaging hand. Reach with your fingertips as far down the back as possible to the lower shoulder muscles.

2 Knead the muscles by squeezing them gently between your fingers and the heel of your hand, applying pressure with the fingertips. Reduce the pressure as your hand begins to slide off the shoulder to prevent the skin being pinched. Repeat the stroke several times. You can increase the pressure if it feels right or you can hold the squeeze for a few seconds instead of sliding your hand off.

DIGITAL EFFLEURAGE – BACK OF THE HEAD

Massage to the base of the skull affects the nerves going up to the head as well as the attachments of the neck muscles.

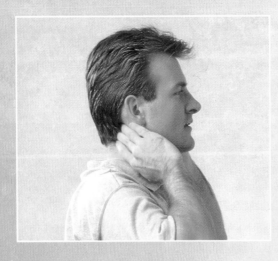
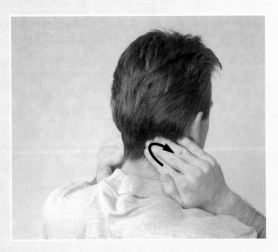

1 Place the fingers at the back of the head underneath the base of the skull. Apply pressure with the fingertips in small circles.

2 Repeat this digital effleurage all along the base of the skull. This area may be very tender, so adjust the pressure accordingly.

ACUPRESSURE POINTS

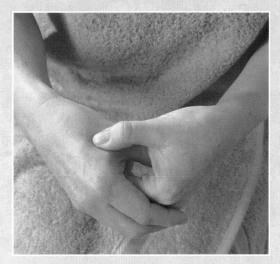

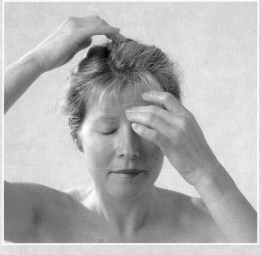

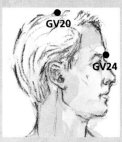

Acupressure points can be used to help ease tension headache. Combine them with the self-administered massage techniques, either following the digital effleurage to the back of the head or following the scalp massage.

Point Hoku (LI 4) Press gently for a few seconds with the thumb of the treating hand. **Location:** in the web between the thumb and first finger. This point should not be stimulated during pregnancy.

Third eye and **Top of head:** Apply gentle pressure on these points while sitting. Work on them simultaneously. Hold the pressure for a few seconds. **Location:** Between the eyebrows and at the centre of the head respectively.

SCALP MASSAGE

1 Use the fingertips to apply pressure and to move the scalp over the skull in small circles. Do not let your fingers slide over the skin. Start at the temples, just above the ears, then cover the top and then the back of the head. Massage each area for a few minutes. The whole sequence can be repeated once more if it feels appropriate.

Tension headaches are reduced by this movement, which helps to ease congestion of blood, nerves and muscle tissue in the scalp.

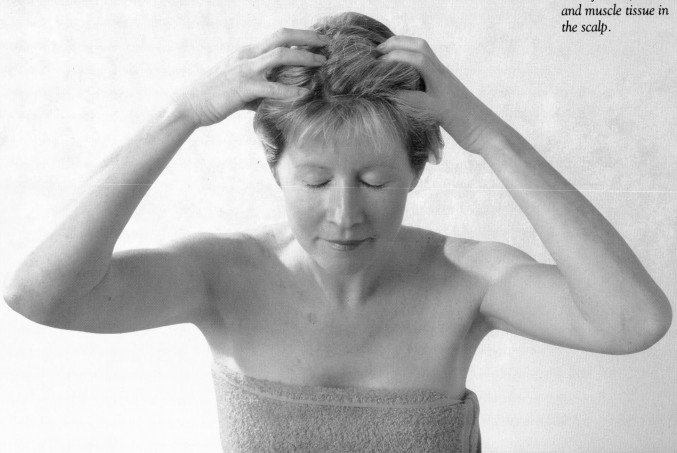

3

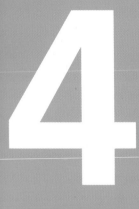

RELAXATION

Reducing stress and achieving relaxation is a difficult task for some people. It is a vital task nonetheless judging by the growing number of stress related conditions. Massage, combined with other forms of relaxation such as meditation and visualization, is perhaps one of the best ways of achieving this goal.

Stress can be described as an overloading of the body's resources which are used to deal with demands made by physical, mental, emotional and environmental factors. The body is capable of adapting to certain levels of stress. Competitive sports, for example, create a certain amount of tension. This is normally welcomed by competitors because they enjoy the "adrenaline buzz" feeling it brings. In more threatening circumstances, however, the body adapts by altering behavioural patterns. These can be minor, like those seen when someone is "on edge" and "jittery", or more serious, like obsessions and eccentricity.

The body also adapts to stress by changing its own physical functions. Muscular tension is a very good example. It is an involuntary reaction by the body so we have no control over it. What is more, even after the stress factors are removed, the physical adaptation by the body may continue. This is why the long-term outcome of stress can be heart disease.

Recognizing the stress patterns in our lives and learning how to deal with them may go some way to preventing disease. How we do this, and the changes we make in our lives is a matter of information, awareness and choice. Somewhere along the line there is also a place for relaxation methods like visualization and massage.

RELAXATION

To counteract stress you need concentration. This may sound contradictory because tension itself can be the result of too much concentration. However, it is also true to say that to "switch off" from one thing you need to concentrate on another. This focusing on a single object, thought or concept gives us the basis of relaxation.

MEDITATION

To focus on one thought or image you need to push aside all other thoughts and images. This is done on a conscious level but without any forceful intention. As a new image or thought comes to the fore you must gently push it aside and return to the main object of concentration. This is a form of exercise which takes some time to perfect. At the beginning, and until you perfect the technique, other thoughts and images will take over very rapidly and quite frequently. You will therefore lose your point of focus. Most times you will not be aware of it happening. You will just suddenly find that you have lost your focus point and are thinking of something completely different. This is a normal process for a mind which is not able to settle down to one thought due to the other worrying thoughts around. The object of the exercise is to train the mind to focus on the one thought and let go of all others. This is the principle of meditation.

EXERCISES FOR RELAXATION

The following techniques are exercises which help focus the mind on one thought. I call them exercises because you need to practise them on a regular basis before you begin to get their full benefit. If you find that you have lost your focus point during the exercise try to return to it gently without any extreme effort. There may be times when you drop off to sleep during such an exercise. This happens if you relax too deeply and too quickly. It is not wrong in itself, but as you develop the technique you will be able to relax without sleeping. On the other hand, as I shall explain later on, you can also use some of these techniques to help you drift off to sleep. These exercises are done sitting or lying down.

BREATHING

One of the easiest ways of relaxing is to concentrate on the breathing. As a result of tension or habit breathing tends to be very short and shallow – with this exercise we aim to change this pattern.

Close your eyes and begin to be aware of your breathing. Follow the breath in and out. Try to increase the length and depth of your in-breath without making too much of an effort. You may feel slight dizziness due to an increase in oxygen to the brain. This is perfectly normal, but if it happens breathe normally for a few moments and it will disappear. The rhythm of the breathing is very important in all forms of relaxation. The slower it is the more relaxed the body gets. As you become increasingly aware of your breathing rhythm aim to slow it down by counting as you breathe in and out. The breathing in is usually shorter than the breathing out. For example, you may breathe in to a count of six and breathe out to a count of eight. Use the counting to help you breathe deeply and slowly. It can also be used as a focusing point.

You can meditate in a chair or sitting on the floor. Make sure that you are comfortable. It is easier to concentrate if you close your eyes.

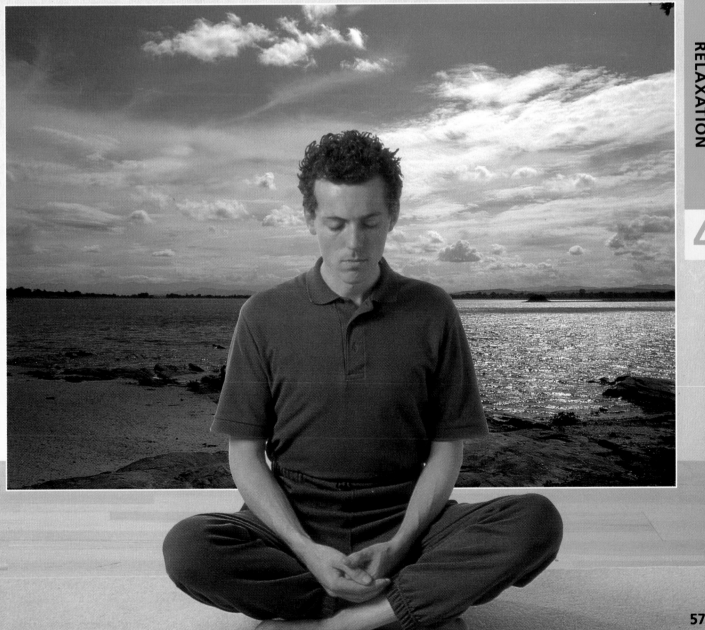

VISUALIZATION

Visualization is another very effective method of relaxation. It can accompany the breathing exercise or be practised as an alternative technique. As well as concentrating on your breathing you can visualize the breath as having a colour as you breathe in. It may be a calm and relaxing colour like a sky blue, or a healing colour like gold, white or amber. You don't need to visualize the out-breath as any particular colour, or you may build up too complicated a picture. On the other hand, you can visualize the out-breath taking with it tension, anxiety, worry and even pain. It is very relaxing to visualize the muscles of the neck and shoulders letting go of tension with each out-breath. Extend this to visualizing the leg muscles relaxing, then the arms, and so on until the whole body lets go. This routine may have to be repeated several times. Do not try to feel the muscles relaxing, just visualize them letting go.

Visualization can take you on many wonderful journeys. The image of a picturesque landscape on a beautiful day, with a blue sky, soft white clouds, rolling hills, flowers blooming and birds singing will help you relax. You can take time building up this picture, visualizing every

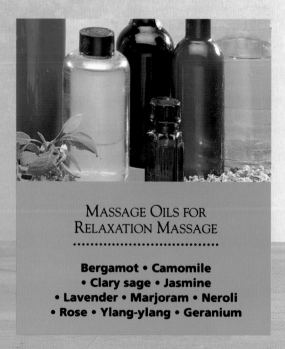

MASSAGE OILS FOR RELAXATION MASSAGE

Bergamot • Camomile • Clary sage • Jasmine • Lavender • Marjoram • Neroli • Rose • Ylang-ylang • Geranium

detail from the shapes of the clouds to the sound of the birds. You can change the place from session to session. The longer you stay with each picture during a session the more relaxing is its effect.

INSOMNIA

Being unable to sleep may be related to anxiety, but the causes of sleeplessness are numerous. For example, the mind needs to reflect and mull over the events of the day. Often we do not allow time for this reflection to happen, and the only time left for the mind to carry out this process is when we are in bed. Allocating time, perhaps during a warm leisurely bath, for reflection before going to bed may prevent insomnia. Bath oils may help, too. Visualization or focusing helps the mind to switch off unnecessary thoughts and drift into sleep. The image may be of a pleasant place, as described earlier, or of an object which has no emotional associations. For example, visualize a flower, then another and another, until you have the image of a beautiful bouquet. The image can be repeated, or another one built up. As you create the image, try to concentrate ever more deeply on its minute and intricate details. Another example which is simple to achieve is that of playing cards being lined up in various patterns according to their numbers, colours or suits. Choose a pattern, and visualize each card being laid down and eventually building up a picture. Many variations of shapes, numbers and colours can be devised for visualization.

MASSAGE

When you use massage for relaxation you have to bear in mind two main points. One is the rhythm of the movements – the slower the movement, the more relaxing the effect. The second is the pressure: light pressure is very relaxing but this does not mean a heavier pressure may not be given during a relaxing massage. As the recipient and their muscles relax, the pressure may be increased as long as it is comfortable.

CREATING THE ATMOSPHERE

The environment for the massage should be quiet and warm. Overhead lighting should be avoided; telephones switched off. Pleasant music – whether classical or popular – helps tremendously to create a relaxed atmosphere, and there are many suitable tapes available. A hot bath, sauna or jacuzzi is a useful start to the process of relaxation.

MASSAGE ROUTINE

There is no set routine for this kind of massage. The recipient may prefer to start with the back or the face. What is important is that the massage "flows", which means that one movement goes smoothly on to the next, and the treatment progresses seamlessly from one area of the body to another. For example, when massaging the back the effleurage techniques follow on from one another without a pause. When the massage starts with the face, the movements follow on to the arms, the abdomen and then the legs. The art of massage involves carrying out the movements in a flowing routine as well as feeling the tissues and adjusting the pressure. It can only come with practice.

This chapter describes a relaxing massage sequence starting with the back. Some of the techniques are illustrated in other chapters but they can easily be incorporated into this routine once the rhythm and pressure of each stroke is adjusted to suit the purpose of relaxation.

DURATION OF THE MASSAGE

The duration of a massage treatment depends on the time available and the area of the body being worked on. A back massage, for example, can take 20 to 30 minutes. The whole body can take between 60 and 90 minutes. Select a routine and techniques to suit your needs.

RELAXATION
Lying down
ROUTINE ONE

Massage to the back

Palm effleurage –
•
Criss-cross effleurage
•
Palm effleurage upper back and shoulders –
•
Thumb effleurage –
•
Kneading –
•
Pick-up effleurage –
•
Reversed palm effleurage
•
Light touch effleurage

Massage to the back of legs

Effleurage – back of leg
•
Thumb effleurage – sole of foot

Massage to the face

Finger effleurage – forehead
•
Pinching pressure – eyebrows
•
Finger effleurage – cheeks
•
Finger effleurage – upper lip and chin
•
Thumb effleurage – ears
•
Fingertip effleurage – cheeks

continued

continued

Palming of the eyes

Supporting hold

Massage to the chest and abdomen

Reversed palm effleurage – chest and abdomen
•
Criss-cross effleurage – abdomen
•
Palm effleurage – abdomen and chest

Massage to the arm

Effleurage – arm
•
Effleurage – hand

Massage to the front of legs

Palm effleurage
•
Effleurage foot

Stillness technique

Acupressure

Reflexology

RELAXATION
Sitting
ROUTINE TWO

Massage to the head and shoulders

Palm effleurage – neck and shoulders
•
Thumb effleurage – upper back / shoulders
•
Kneading – upper back / shoulders
•
Pick-up effleurage – neck

Massage to the face

Effleurage – forehead
•
Pinching eyebrows
•
Effleurage – forehead
•
Effleurage – cheeks
•
Effleurage – upper lip/chin
•
Scalp massage
•
Palming of the eyes

Massage to the arm

Effleurage – arm
•
Effleurage – hand

Massage to the foot

Effleurage

Reflexology

Acupressure

RELAXATION

4

THE BACK

. . . .

This relaxation routine starts with massage to the back and finishes with the stillness technique. The whole sequence lasts about 90 minutes, but you can also select techniques to suit yourself. The recipient is lying down.

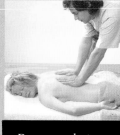

. . . .

CRISS-CROSS EFFLEURAGE

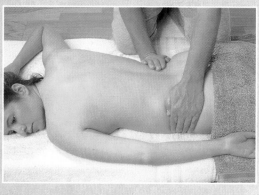
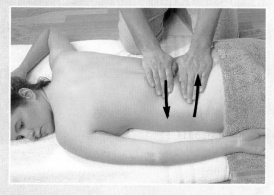

1 *This technique follows palm effleurage.* Position yourself to the side of the recipient. Place both hands on the lower back, one hand on each side of the spine with the fingers pointing away from you.

2 The hands travel in opposite directions, passing close to each other as they effleurage back and forth across the back.

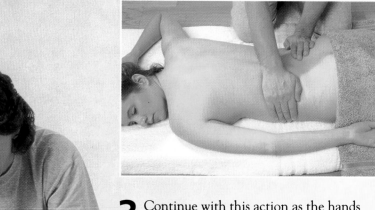

Repeat technique
. . . .
PALM EFFLEURAGE
– BACK
See page 18
•
Before
CRISS–CROSS
EFFLEURAGE

3 Continue with this action as the hands travel upwards towards the head. Include the shoulders and then work the hands down the back again. Repeat the whole sequence.

4 The same technique can be applied across the buttocks. The hands pass each other as they effleurage backwards and forwards. The pressure is applied as each hand travels towards the midline and eases off completely as they travel outwards.

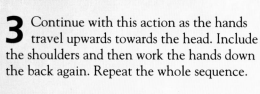

REPEAT TECHNIQUES

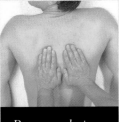

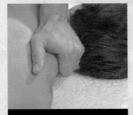

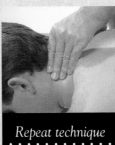

Repeat technique

PALM EFFLEURAGE –
UPPER BACK AND
SHOULDERS
See page 36
•
Follows
CRISS–CROSS
EFFLEURAGE

Repeat technique

THUMB EFFLEURAGE
– UPPER BACK AND
SHOULDERS
See page 40
•
Follows
PALM EFFLEURAGE
– UPPER BACK AND
SHOULDERS

Repeat technique

KNEADING
– UPPER BACK AND
SHOULDERS
See page 45
•
Follows
THUMB EFFLEURAGE
– UPPER BACK AND
SHOULDERS

Repeat technique

PICK-UP EFFLEURAGE
– NECK
See page 46
•
Follows
KNEADING
– UPPER BACK AND
SHOULDERS

REVERSED PALM EFFLEURAGE

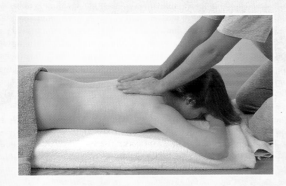

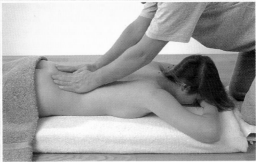

Reversed palm effleurage follows the techniques carried out to individual areas of the back. The slow rhythm induces relaxation.

1 Position yourself at the head of the recipient.

2 Effleurage down the back, one hand on either side of the spine, to the lower back or buttocks (or as far as you can reach comfortably).

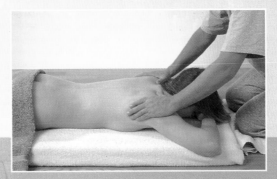

3 When the hands reach the lower back, move them towards the sides of the body and effleurage lightly up towards the shoulders.

4 The effleurage continues over the top of the shoulders and the neck area. As the hands reach the top of the neck the pressure is reduced and the hands lifted off. Repeat the stroke starting from the top of the back.

Position yourself at the side of the recipient. Ideally, this movement should be carried out at the end of the back sequence.

LIGHT-TOUCH EFFLEURAGE

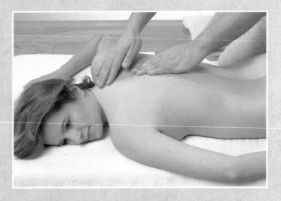

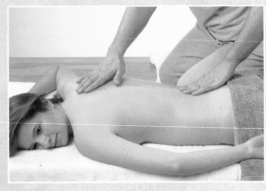

1 Starting with the hands placed at the top end of the back, stroke gently with alternate hands down to the base of the spine. The pressure should be extremely light.

2 When one hand reaches the lower back or buttocks it is lifted off slowly and returned to the top of the back again.

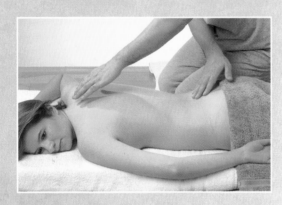

3 The hands follow each other with the effleurage stroke. As one is lifted off the lower back the other starts the next stroke from the top. Repeat for several minutes.

BACK OF LEGS

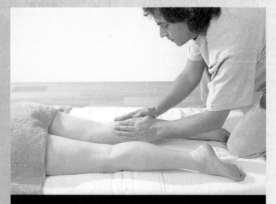

Repeat technique

PALM EFFLEURAGE – BACK OF LEG
See page 125

Follows LIGHT TOUCH EFFLEURAGE – BACK

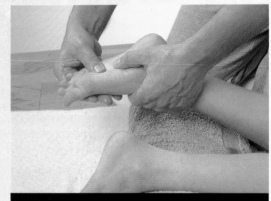

Repeat technique

THUMB EFFLEURAGE – SOLE OF FOOT
See page 147

Follows PALM EFFLEURAGE – BACK OF LEG

THE FACE

. . . .

For the following techniques the recipient lies face upwards.

. . . .

FINGER EFFLEURAGE – ACROSS FOREHEAD

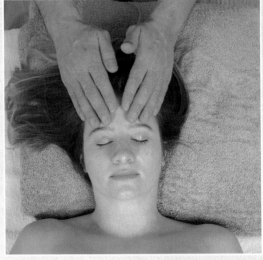

1 With the fingers of each hand pointing towards the feet and placed next to each other on the centre of the forehead, effleurage lightly and gently towards the temples. Use the pads along the length of the fingers and keep each finger straight.

Facial massage is done at this point in the sequence, or at the beginning of the relaxation massage routine. It can also be done separately on its own.

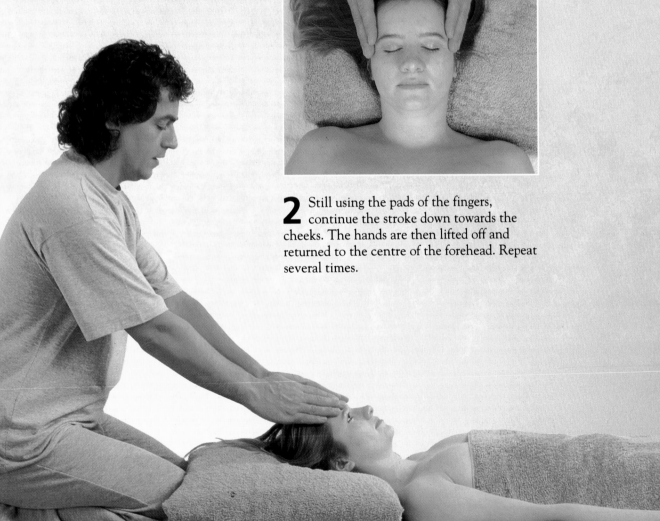

2 Still using the pads of the fingers, continue the stroke down towards the cheeks. The hands are then lifted off and returned to the centre of the forehead. Repeat several times.

PINCHING PRESSURE MOVEMENT – ACROSS EYEBROWS

This technique is used both for relaxation and for sinus congestion, as it affects a number of reflex points located here.

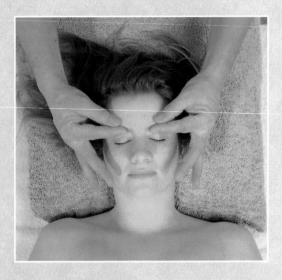

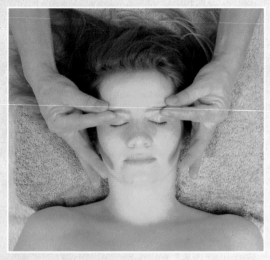

1 With the thumb and first finger of each hand pinch the eyebrows gently at their inner ends and hold for a few seconds.

2 Release the pressure and move the hands a little way towards the temples. Apply the pinching pressure and then move once more. Repeat all along the eyebrows.

FLAT FINGER EFFLEURAGE – ACROSS CHEEKS

Effleurage to the cheeks is relaxing and helps with the lymphatic drainage in the area.

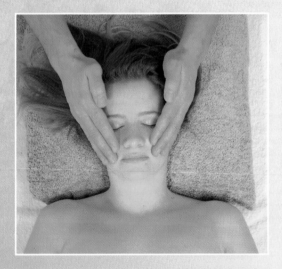

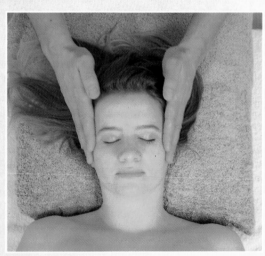

1 Using flat fingers, effleurage the cheeks, starting from the sides of the nose and working towards the ears.

2 As the fingers reach the ears they continue the effleurage on the sides of the face and neck. They are then lifted off and the movement repeated several times.

FLAT FINGERS EFFLEURAGE – ACROSS UPPER LIP AND CHIN

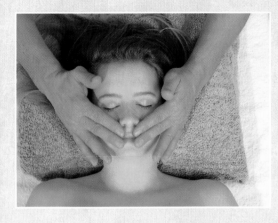

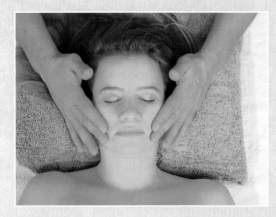

Like the previous movement this has a relaxing effect, as well as enhancing lymphatic drainage.

1 Effleurage across the upper lip with the first and second fingers. Start from the centre and continue as far as the cheeks.

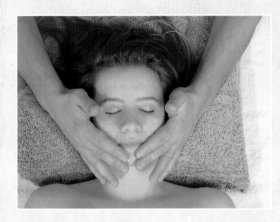

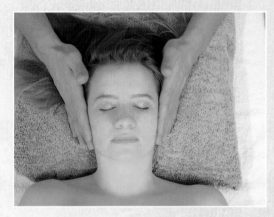

2 The same fingers are used to effleurage the chin, starting from the middle and working outwards towards the jaw. Keep the fingers flat and the pressure light.

3 At the jaw the hands turn, to point towards the chest, so as to effleurage down the sides of the neck.

THUMB EFFLEURAGE – EARS

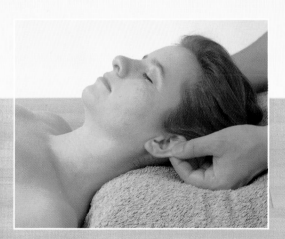

1 Both ears are massaged together. Support each ear with the fingertips. Use the thumbs to apply pressure in very small circles on the fleshy part of the ears, and work the thumbs around the outside of each ear. There is no need to repeat this movement.

Several reflex points relating to the whole body are located around the ears, and therefore massaging the area has a very beneficial effect, as well as being relaxing.

FINGERTIP EFFLEURAGE – ACROSS CHEEKS

Massage to the cheek-bones helps with sinus congestion. This is because several reflex points are located there. In addition, it enhances lymphatic drainage.

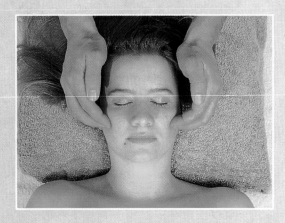

1 Curve the fingers slightly so the fingertips can apply pressure just underneath the cheekbone. Start from the centre near the nose and work outwards as far as the ear. Repeat several times.

PALMING – OF EYES

Apply this technique as part of the facial massage sequence, or at the end of the whole body massage routine.

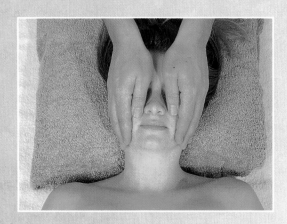

1 Place both hands on top of the closed eyes. Covering the eyes with the hands may feel slightly threatening to start with, but as the recipient gets used to it the palming becomes very relaxing. No pressure is applied other than the weight of the hands. Hold the position for a few minutes. Both hands must be kept very relaxed and free of tension.

SUPPORTING HOLD

This is not strictly speaking a massage technique but it is included in this routine because of its relaxing effect. Holding the head in this manner is emotionally supportive and encourages the recipient to let go of tension.

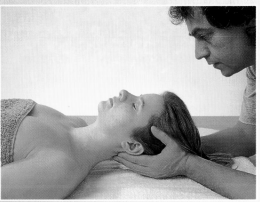

Take care not to:

Apply this technique to someone during a migraine attack as it could worsen the symptoms

•

Some people may find it uncomfortable to hold this position for more than a few minutes if they suffer from certain conditions like arthritis of the neck

1 First settle into a comfortable position at the head of the recipient. Place your hands together on the floor or massage plinth with the palms turned up. The recipient then rests his or her head on your hands. Encourage him or her to let go of the weight of the head and to let it sink further into your palms. Ask him or her to take a few deep breaths and to "let go" on each out-breath. When you feel the recipient has settled down, hold this position for a few minutes to induce further relaxation.

CHEST AND ABDOMEN

The chest and abdomen are perhaps the most vulnerable areas of the body so ensure that the strokes and pressure are acceptable to the recipient.

REVERSED PALM EFFLEURAGE – CHEST AND ABDOMEN

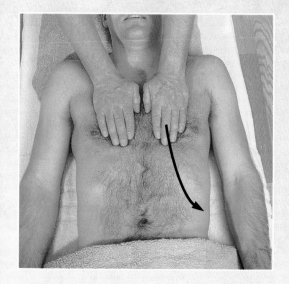

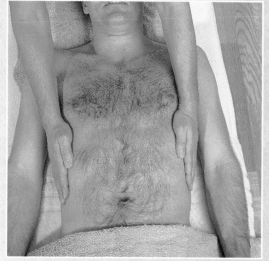

Apply this technique as a starting movement for the chest and abdomen. It can also be repeated after the other strokes.

1 Position yourself at the head of the recipient. Place your hands centrally on the top of the chest and begin to effleurage down towards the abdomen. When massaging a woman the hands move close together between the breasts. If it is difficult to reach the abdominal area take the hands down as far as you can comfortably reach.

2 Continue the stroke towards the sides of the body, maintaining the same pressure, but not pressing heavily on the abdominal region. Now, effleurage upwards on the sides of the trunk towards the shoulders.

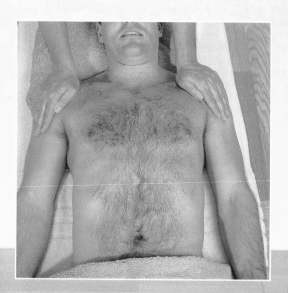

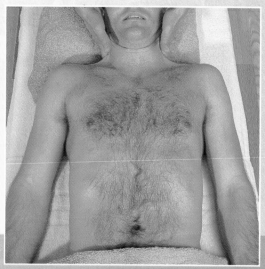

3 Continue the effleurage over the shoulders moulding the hands to their contours.

4 The movement ends as the hands travel underneath the neck to the base of the skull. Return the hands to the chest and repeat the movement.

RELAXATION

4

CRISS-CROSS EFFLEURAGE – ABDOMEN

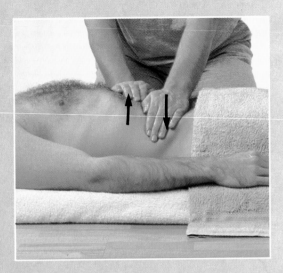

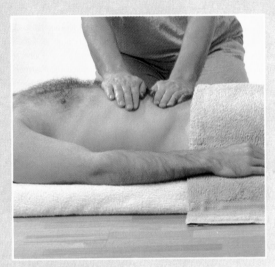

*This technique helps
to relax the muscles
and increases
abdominal and
body temperature.*

1 Position yourself beside the recipient.
Place your hands on the abdomen.
Effleurage by moving your hands back and
forth past each other. Keep your hands close
together all the time.

2 With the same stroke work upwards
towards the chest and downwards towards
the pubic area. Ensure that the movement is
comfortable to the recipient at all times. The
rhythm should be very slow.

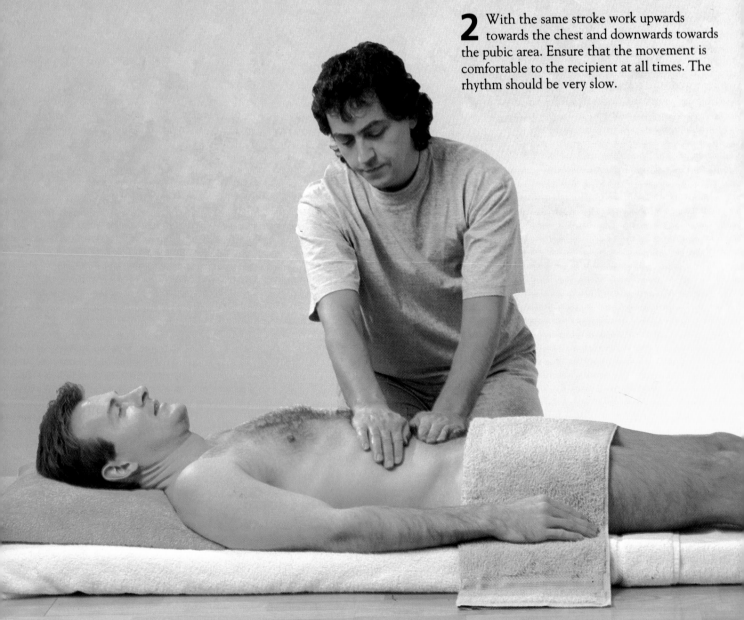

PALM EFFLEURAGE – ABDOMEN AND CHEST

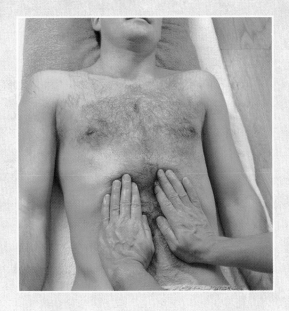

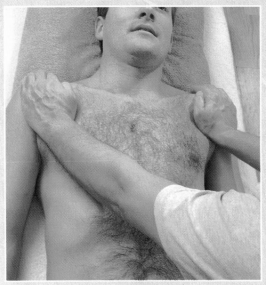

Try to create a rhythm for each stroke. This is a very relaxing movement when carried out very slowly and with light pressure.

1 Starting at the abdominal area effleurage with the palms of both hands from the abdomen and over the chest towards the head. When massaging a woman the hands move close together between the breasts. The hands can also be lifted off to avoid the breast tissue altogether.

2 As you reach the top of the chest move your hands towards and over the shoulders. Cup your hands as you go over the shoulders and increase the pressure slightly.

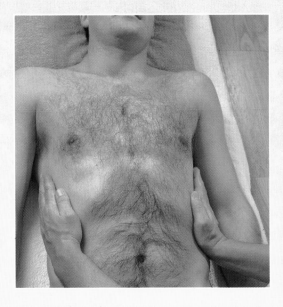

3 Continue the stroke on the sides of the trunk towards the pelvis. At waist level turn the hands so the fingers point towards the sides of the trunk and stroke towards the centre of the abdomen. Position the hands with the fingertips pointing towards the head and repeat the movement several times.

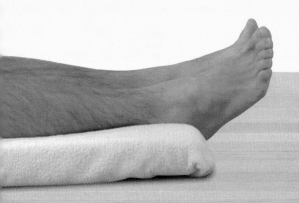

RELAXATION

4

69

THE ARM

Repeat the massage strokes to the arm and hand several times. Adjust the position of the arm so that you can carry out the movements comfortably.

EFFLEURAGE – ARM

This effleurage helps to increase circulation to the hands when the emphasis is on the stroke towards the hand (Step 3).

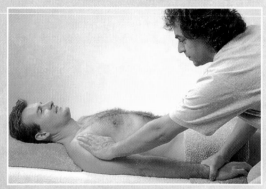

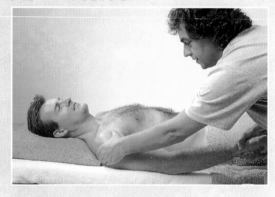

1 With one hand hold the recipient's wrist, and with the other effleurage up the arm. Keep the palm and fingers straight but relaxed.

2 Cup the hand to go over the shoulder.

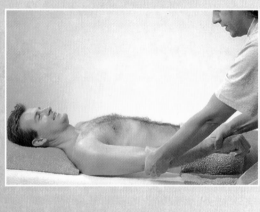

3 Gently squeeze the arm between your fingers and thumb as you effleurage down towards the hand.

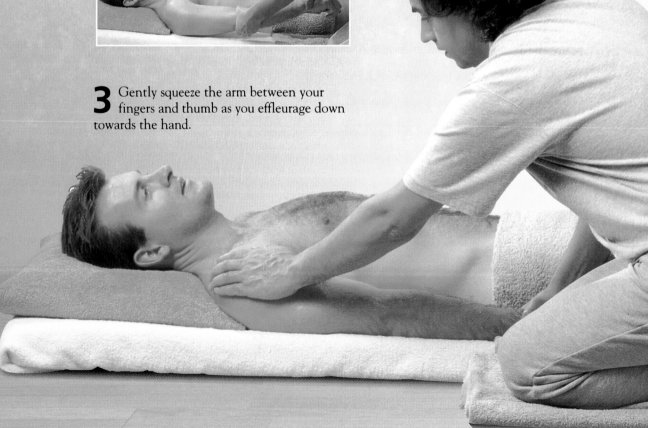

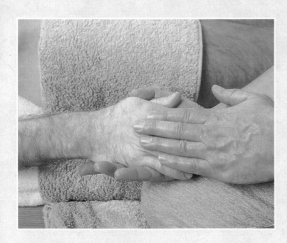

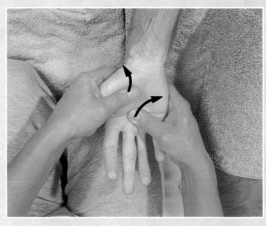

Apart from being very relaxing, massage to the hands also works on reflex points related to the whole body.

1 Using the palm and fingers of one hand, effleurage the back of the recipient's hand several times.

2 Turn the hand palm upwards, and using your thumbs effleurage in small circles all over the palm.

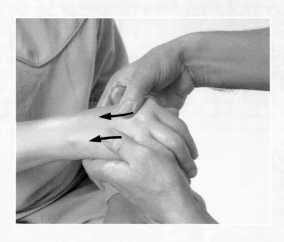

3 Use the thumbs to effleurage the back of the hand and wrist. Support the recipient's hand with both of yours. Apply a semi-circular stroke with each thumb alternately. Use firm pressure and continue the movement for a minute or so.

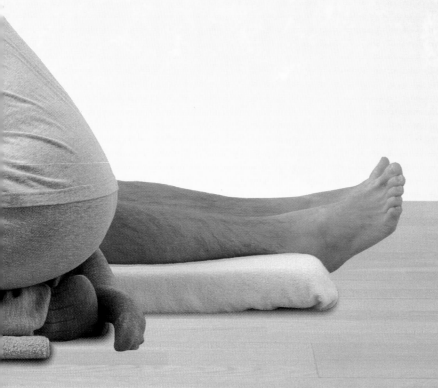

RELAXATION

4

THE LEG

The techniques on the leg and the foot are carried out with medium pressure and a slow rhythm for general relaxation. The upstroke enhances the venous return and the down stroke increases circulation to the foot.

PALM EFFLEURAGE – FRONT OF LEG

This effleurage starts at the ankle and works up to the top of the leg, so position yourself where you can comfortably reach both.

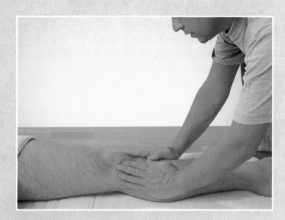

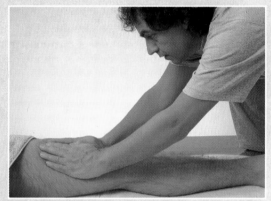

1 Place the hands so as to cover as much of the roundness of the leg as possible. Start with the hands covering the inner and outer aspects of the lower leg. When the stroke is repeated they are moved to another area so that all of the inner, outer and top regions are massaged. Be careful not to press on the shin bone. Continue the effleurage towards the thigh. Care should be taken so that no pressure is applied over the knee.

2 When you reach the top of the thigh take the outer hand to the outer border and the inner to the inner border of the thigh.

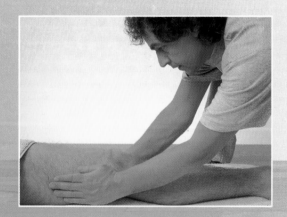

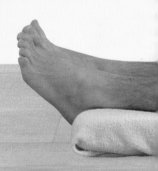

3 Return with a very light effleurage as the hands run down to the ankle for the movement to be repeated.

EFFLEURAGE – FOOT

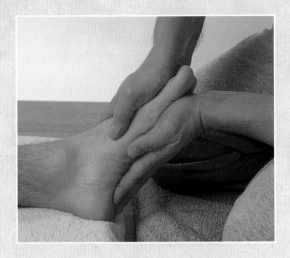

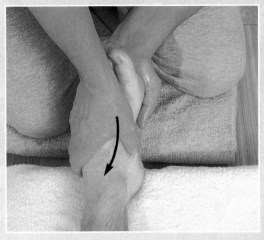

Some people find massage to the foot more relaxing than that to any other area of the body, while others may find the feet too ticklish to be touched.

1 Use one hand to support the sole of the foot while the second massages the top part of it.

2 Effleurage with the palm and fingers, starting at the toes and working towards the ankle, finishing with the thumb on the inside and the fingers on the outside of the ankle.

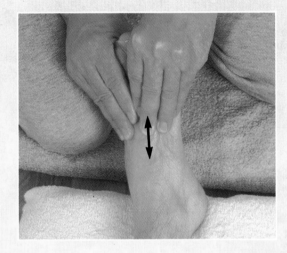

STILLNESS TECHNIQUE

The solar plexus is situated in the centre of an imaginary line which divides the chest and the abdomen. Place one hand over the recipient's solar plexus area, very lightly, without any pressure whatsoever. Place the second hand on the forehead, keeping the pressure as light as possible. Hold this position for a few minutes to encourage deep relaxation. You must be in a relaxed state yourself, so you may find it helpful to do some relaxation breathing.

3 A second effleurage to the foot can be done mostly with the fingertips positioned on the top of the foot and the thumbs underneath. Applying a firm pressure, the fingers travel forwards and backwards on one area before moving to another, still on the top of the foot.

ACUPRESSURE POINTS

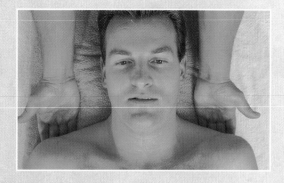

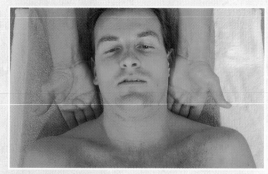

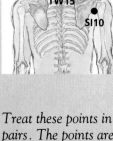

TW15: Slightly above the top corner of the shoulder blade nearest to the spine.

GB21: This point is found on the top of the shoulder, halfway between the base of the neck and the shoulder joint. As this is usually a lumpy area associated with muscle tension it is not difficult to locate.

Treat these points in pairs. The points are illustrated with the recipient lying face upwards. They can also be treated with the recipient lying face downwards.

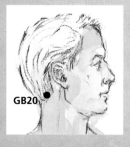

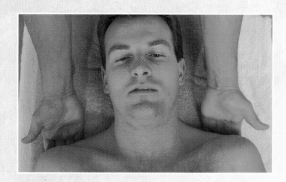

GB20: On each side of the spine, halfway between the spine and the bony prominence behind the ear. There is a tiny hollow in between two groups of muscles at the base of the skull (occiput) in the central area where this point is located.

SI10: This point is found along the outer edge of the scapula (shoulder blade) just below the point where it meets the humerus (upper arm bone). Another way of describing this location is at the back of the axilla (armpit) just below the shoulder joint.

Top of head and Third eye: Each of these is a single central point, and they are treated together as a pair. Mid-cervical and GB14: Treat these points together on one side of the body and then repeat on the other side.

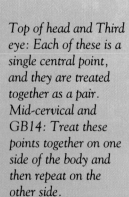

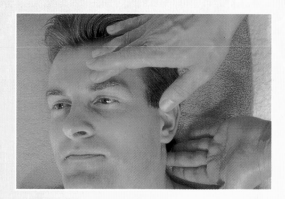

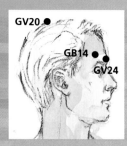

Top of head (GV20): At the very centre of the top of the head.
Third eye (GV24): On the forehead in between the eyebrows.

Mid-cervical: This is halfway between the base of the skull (occiput) and the lower end of the neck, to the side of the bony prominence. This point tends to be contra-indicated during pregnancy.
GB14: One finger's width above the eyebrows, in line with the centre of the pupil of the eye, in a tiny hollow. Press very gently when treating.

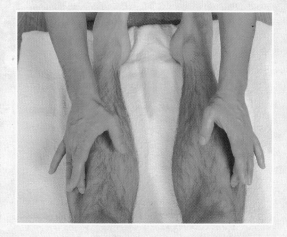

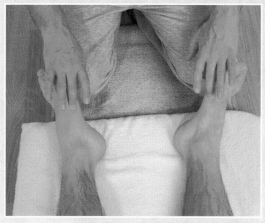

Sanri St36: Position yourself at the feet of the recipient and treat these points as a pair. These points are found on the outer aspects of the lower legs. Locate the two bones of the lower leg, just below the knee joint. One bone is to the front, the tibia and the second one to the outside, the fibula. The acupressure point is located where these two bones meet, just below the knee.

Sp4: Treat as a pair, i.e. on the left and right sides simultaneously. On the inner edge of the foot. From the base of the big toe follow the bone line towards the heel on the inner aspect of the foot. About halfway between the base of the toe and the heel there is a bony prominence. The acupressure point is located just below it towards the sole of the foot. It is often fairly sensitive to pressure.

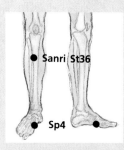

REFLEX POINTS

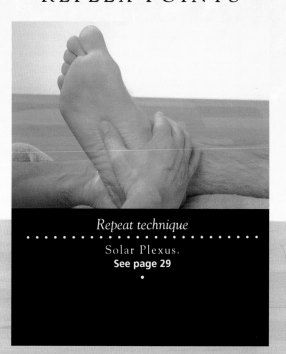

Repeat technique

Solar Plexus.
See page 29
•

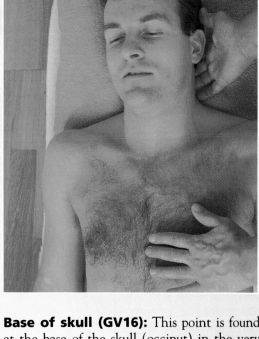

These two points are treated together with one hand on the sternum (breast bone) and the second hand on the base of the skull.

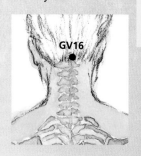

Base of skull (GV16): This point is found at the base of the skull (occiput) in the very centre where it joins the top of the neck.

Centre of sternum (CV17): The sternum runs downwards between the ribs at the front of the chest. Find the midpoint between the top and lower ends of the bone, and the centre of bone across the width, to find this acupressure point.

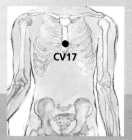

THE HEAD AND SHOULDERS
· ·

A number of the relaxation techniques can be applied with the recipient sitting down. This is a very useful position if the recipient or the giver is unable to work on the floor

· ·

REPEAT TECHNIQUES

The following movements on the neck and shoulders have already been demonstrated. They can be incorpprated into this relaxation routine with the recipient sitting down.

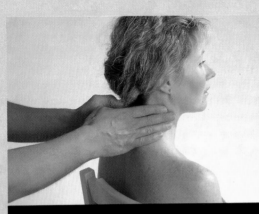

Repeat technique
· ·
PALM EFFLEURAGE – NECK AND SHOULDERS
See page 44
•
Followed by THUMB EFFLEURAGE – UPPER BACK AND SHOULDERS

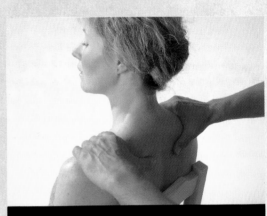

Repeat technique
· ·
THUMB EFFLEURAGE – UPPER BACK AND SHOULDERS
See page 45
•
Followed by KNEADING – UPPER BACK AND SHOULDERS

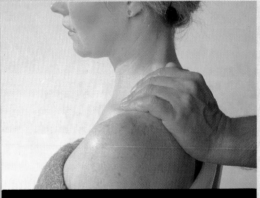

Repeat technique
· ·
KNEADING – UPPER BACK AND SHOULDERS
See page 45
•
Followed by PICK-UP EFFLEURAGE – NECK

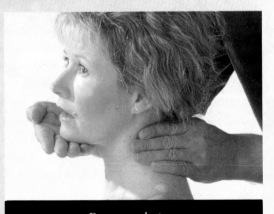

Repeat technique
· ·
PICK-UP EFFLEURAGE – NECK
See page 46
•
Followed by FLAT FINGERS EFFLEURAGE – ACROSS FOREHEAD

THE FACE

*Facial massage is very relaxing and can be done separately as a routine on its own.
Here, it is incorporated in the general massage routine.*

FLAT FINGERS EFFLEURAGE – ACROSS FOREHEAD

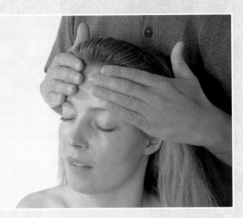

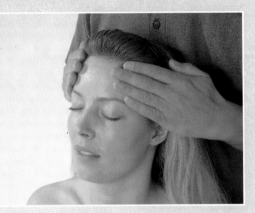

This technique feels as if it is ironing out tension; sometimes noticeable as frown creases on the forehead.

1 Place the hands next to each other on the forehead with the fingers pointing towards each other. Starting from the central area, effleurage gently towards the temples.

2 Once the hands reach the temples the stroke continues down towards the cheeks. The hands are then lifted off and returned to the centre of the forehead. Repeat several times.

PINCHING PRESSURE MOVEMENT – ACROSS EYEBROWS

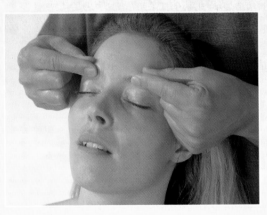

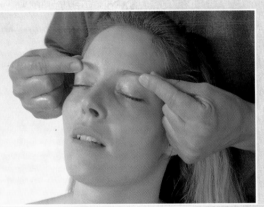

Compression massage technique to the eyebrows is used for relaxation, as well as for sinus congestion since it affects a number of reflex points located here.

1 With the thumbs and first fingers, pinch the eyebrows gently and hold for a few seconds.

2 Release the pressure and move the hands a little way towards the temples. Apply the pinching pressure again before moving. Repeat all along the eyebrow.

FIRST FINGER PRESSURE AND EFFLEURAGE – FOREHEAD

This movement combines a massage stroke with pressure on acupressure points on either side of the nose and the forehead.

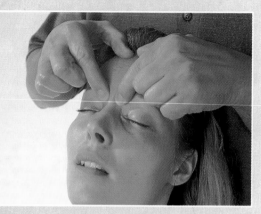 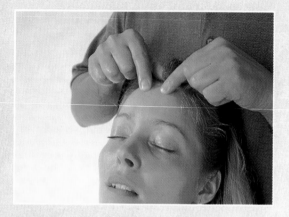

1 Stand behind the recipient and rest the head on your abdomen or chest. You may use a cushion or folded towel under the head. Place the tip of the first finger of each hand on either side of the nose where it meets the eye socket or eyebrows. Apply a gentle pressure there without sliding or moving for about six seconds.

2 Begin to slide the fingertips upwards towards the hairline, applying a slight pressure. When the fingers reach the top of the forehead lift off and return to the first position. Repeat a few times.

FLAT FINGERS EFFLEURAGE – ACROSS CHEEKS

Effleurage to the cheeks is relaxing and helps with the lymphatic drainage in the area.

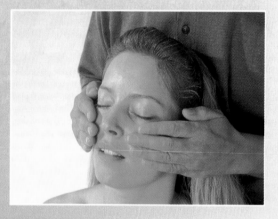 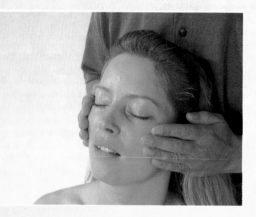

1 Starting from the sides of the nose, using flat fingers, effleurage the cheeks, working towards the ears.

2 As the fingers reach the ears continue the effleurage on the sides of the face and neck. Then lift them off and repeat the movement several times.

FLAT FINGERS EFFLEURAGE – ACROSS UPPER LIP AND CHIN

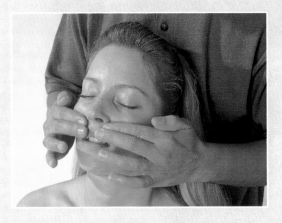

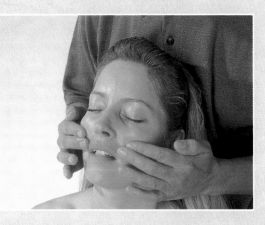

Like the previous movement this has a relaxing effect, as well as enhancing lymphatic drainage.

1 The first and second fingers are used to effleurage across the upper lip, starting from the centre.

2 Continue the effleurage as far as the cheeks before repeating it several times.

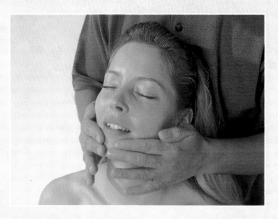

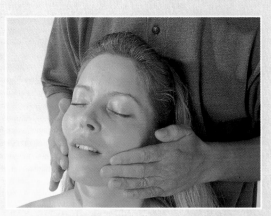

3 Use the same fingers to effleurage the chin starting from the middle and working outwards towards the jaw articulation. Keep the fingers flat and the pressure light.

4 When you reach the jaw articulation turn the hands towards the feet to effleurage down the sides of the neck.

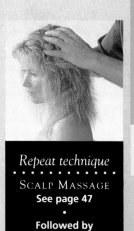

RELAXATION

4

Repeat technique
. . . .
SCALP MASSAGE
See page 47
•
Followed by
PALMING –
OF EYES

PALMING – OF EYES

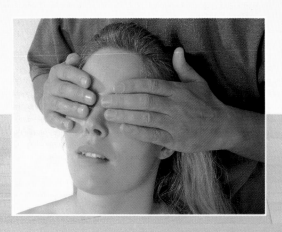

1 *This technique follows scalp massage.*
Ask the recipient to close the eyes and gently rest your hands on them. Covering the eyes in this fashion may feel slightly threatening to start with but as the recipient gets accustomed to it the technique becomes very relaxing. No pressure is applied other than the weight of the hands. Hold the position for a few minutes, keeping both hands very relaxed and free of tension.

THE ARM

Massage strokes to the arm increase the circulation, particularly to the hand, but they are also relaxing when carried out in a slow rhythm.

EFFLEURAGE

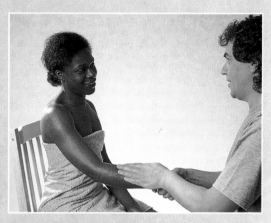

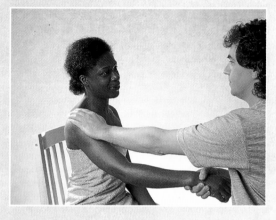

1 Holding the hand of the recipient at the wrist, use your second hand to effleurage the forearm and upper arm. Keep your palm and fingers straight but relaxed.

2 Cup the hand to go over the shoulder.

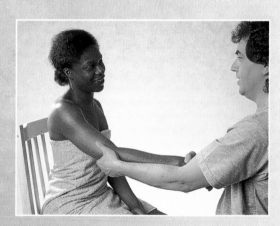

3 Maintain a gentle squeeze between the fingers and the thumb as you effleurage down the arm towards the wrist. Repeat several times.

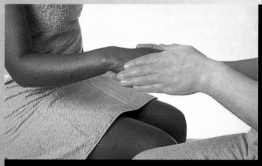

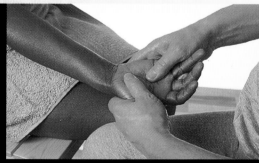

Repeat technique

EFFLEURAGE – HAND
See page 71
•
Follows EFFLEURAGE – ARM

THE FOOT

Massaging the feet can be extremely relaxing, but, on the other hand, it may prove too ticklish.

EFFLEURAGE

RELAXATION

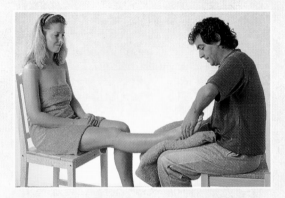

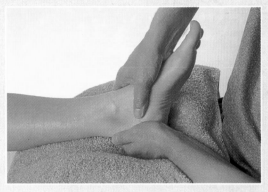

This movement can be carried out with the recipient's foot resting on a cushion placed on your lap.

1 With one hand support the sole of the foot while the second hand massages the top part. Use the palm and fingers to effleurage with.

2 Starting at the toes work towards the ankle, finishing with the thumb on the inside and the fingers on the outside of the ankle.

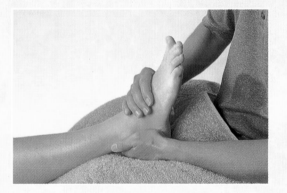

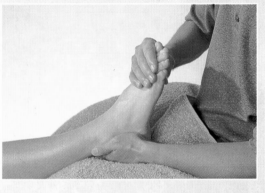

3 Gently squeeze with the flat of your fingers placed across the upper part of the foot and the thumbs underneath.

4 Starting from the heel, squeeze as you slide your hands up towards the toes. Repeat several times.

4

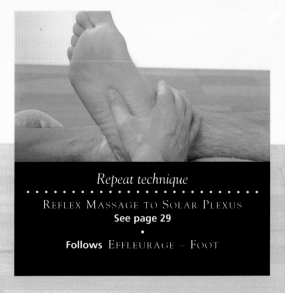

Repeat technique

REFLEX MASSAGE TO SOLAR PLEXUS
See page 29

•

Follows EFFLEURAGE – FOOT

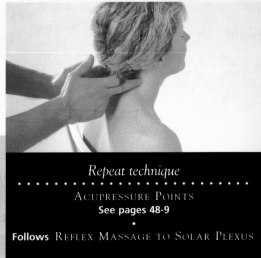

Repeat technique

ACUPRESSURE POINTS
See pages 48-9

•

Follows REFLEX MASSAGE TO SOLAR PLEXUS

5

SPORTS

SPORTS

Massage has a number of applications in the realm of sport. It is used in training, before and after exercise and sporting events, and as part of the rehabilitation regime. Although the techniques are similar, the emphasis is different in each application.

Any exercise can lead to injury if it is not done with care. Muscles, for example, can be easily injured if they are not properly warmed up or if they are overworked. The body can be susceptible to injury due to mechanical imbalances or weaknesses. The repetitive movements of step exercise, for example, may lead to pelvic imbalances or ligament strain.

Before a sporting event the muscles are being warmed up in preparation for intensive work. After the event massage is used to relax the muscles and reduce any build-up of waste products. The rhythm and pressure vary from one situation to the other. Warm-up massage techniques include fast effleurage and percussive strokes; post-exercise strokes include circulation drainage effleurage and petrissage.

WARM-UP PRIOR TO EXERCISE

Warming up before any sporting activity is very important. Stretching and toning helps to reduce the possibility of muscle injury. A muscle works by lengthening and shortening, to varying degrees and at different speeds. This can only be accommodated safely once the tissue within and around the muscle is stretched and warmed up.

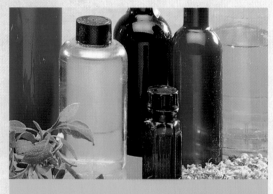

MASSAGE OILS
. . . .

To warm and tone up muscles
Juniper • Black pepper • Rosemary

To reduce muscle spasm
Clary sage • Jasmine • Marjoram

To reduce pain in muscles
Camomile • Lavender • Marjoram

To reduce inflammation and bruising
Camomile • Lavender • Myrrh

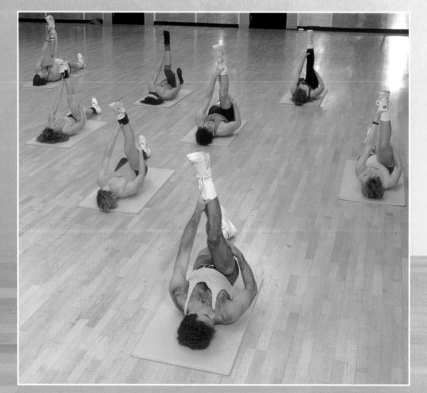

MASSAGE DURING TRAINING

During the training period massage is used to increase the circulation through the muscles and to loosen up the tissues. The increased blood flow provides nutrients and reduces any build-up of lactic acid and carbon dioxide, the waste products of muscle work. Loosening up of the tissues keeps the different layers of muscles free to glide over each other as they contract and stretch, and increases their efficiency. The massage can be given at least once a week, on resting days or when light training only is planned.

TRAINING: LEG MUSCLES

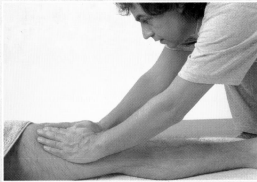

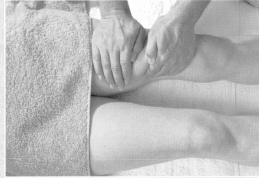

Taking the muscles of the leg as an example the following routine can be followed as a general guide.

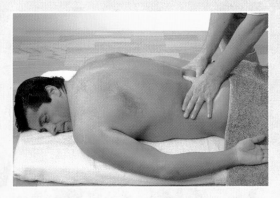

1 **Palm effleurage** to the front of the leg. This is carried out for about five minutes to encourage the circulation towards the heart, thus clearing away toxic materials. The technique has been shown on page 72.

2 Follow the effleurage with **petrissage** to the muscles at the front of the thighs to loosen up the tissues. The technique for the front of the thigh is described on page 122, and for the back of the thigh it is illustrated on page 86.

3 Use **thumb effleurage** to work deep into any "knotted" areas which feel hard and uneven. This has been demonstrated on the lower back on page 18.

4 Repeat the **palm effleurage** for a further few minutes.

5 Repeat the same movements on the back of the leg.

Take care not to:
· · · · · · · · · · ·

Use massage where there is an injury like a muscle strain or bruising. In such situations it is advisable to refer to a qualified sports therapist. See also the advice later on in this chapter.

SPORTS

5

SPORTS ROUTINE **Massage in training**	SPORTS ROUTINE **Massage before sports**	**continued**	SPORTS ROUTINE **Massage after sports**	SPORTS ROUTINE **Self-administered massage** BEFORE SPORTS
Palm effleurage · Petrissage · Thumb effleurage	**Massage to the leg** Brisk effleurage · Crisscross effleurage · Petrissage · Percussive movements: · Little finger strike · Cupping · Flat fist pounding	**Massage to the back** Palm effleurage · Criss-cross effleurage · Percussive movements: · Little finger strike · Cupping **Massage to the arm** Effleurage · Petrissage · Percussive strokes: · Little finger strike · Cupping	**Massage to the leg** Effleurage · Lymph drainage · Petrissage **Massage to the back** Effleurage	**Massage to the leg** Palm effleurage · Alternating palm effleurage · Criss-cross effleurage **Following sports** Effleurage to leg

MASSAGE FOR WARMING UP – THE LEG

Massage is used along with stretching exercises and other warm-up techniques just prior to a sporting activity to warm up the muscles. It is most beneficial given 15 minutes or so before the activity. The following are some of the techniques which can be employed. They are carried out on the legs and arms most of the time although the back muscles can also be included if necessary. However, they are only of benefit if the recipient does not get cold prior to, during and straight after the massage.

BRISK EFFLEURAGE

Apply the warm up effleurage to the front, as well as to the back, of the leg.

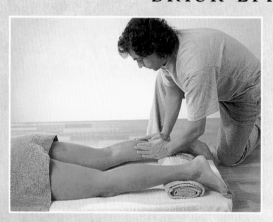

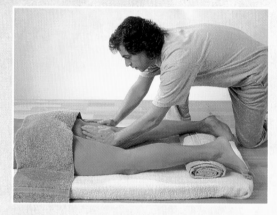

1 The warm-up routine always starts with a brisk effleurage. The hands travel from the ankle upwards towards the pelvis, and should be curved around the leg to cover as much area as possible. The strokes should be fairly brisk and the pressure firm but not heavy.

2 When the hands reach the top of the thigh the outer hand moves to the outer border and the inner hand to the inside of the thigh.

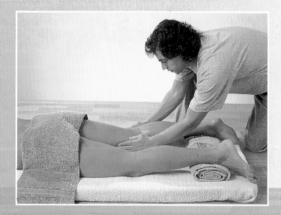

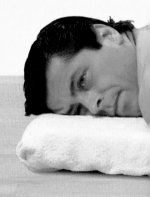

3 Effleurage lightly down to the ankle again and repeat the stroke several times.

CRISS-CROSS EFFLEURAGE

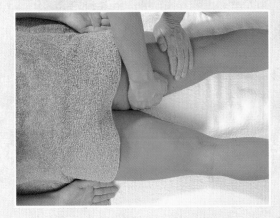

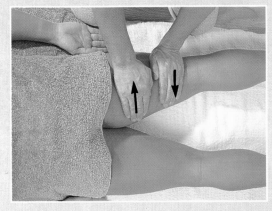

This technique can be applied on most muscle groups and is especially suitable for those at the front and back of the thigh and for the calf muscles.

1 Position yourself to the side of the recipient (see below). Place both hands on top of the thigh, one on the outer and one on the inner region, the fingers pointing away from you.

2 Effleurage across the thigh as the hands travel towards each other.

3 Repeat the criss-cross movement along the whole length of the thigh. Use very brisk movements to warm up the tissues.

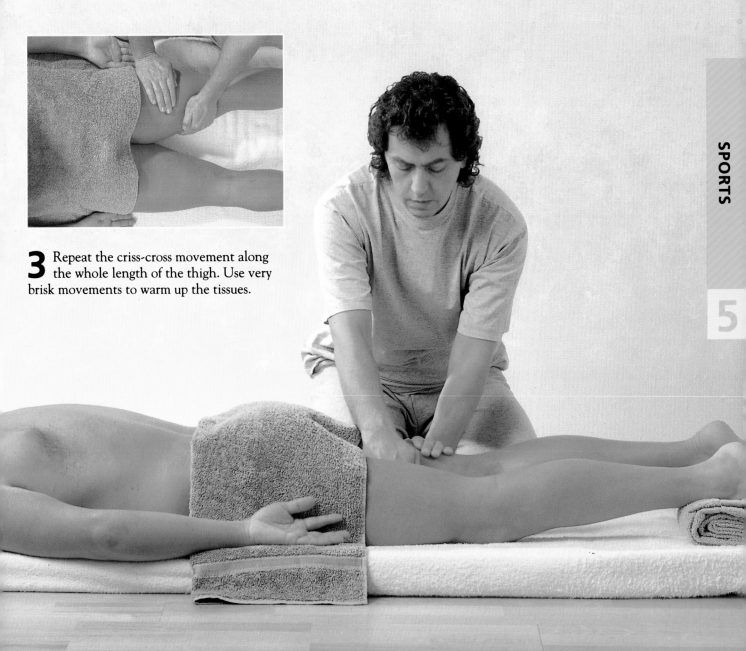

5

PETRISSAGE

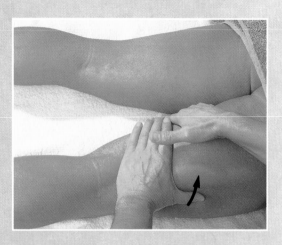

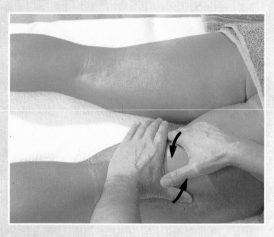

Petrissage lifts the muscle groups away from the underlying bone while compressing the muscle tissue. It takes a little time to master, but once this is achieved it is very pleasant and effective. The technique is also applied to the front thigh muscle.

1 Place the fingers of one hand on the inside of the muscles at the back of the thigh. The heel of the other hand is placed on the outside.

2 Lift and compress the muscle groups by applying pressure with both hands. Continue with the compression but let your hands slide towards the centre. Add a gentle twist of the tissues at the same time.

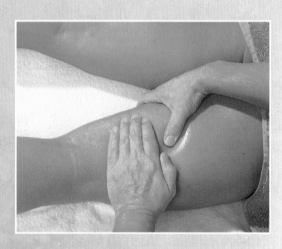

3 Reduce the pressure as the muscle bulk slips away from your grip. Be careful not to pinch the skin. Repeat the movement so that each hand alternately starts on the inside of the thigh, working up and down the length of the thigh.

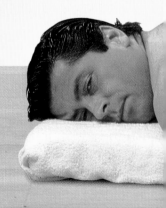

PERCUSSIVE MOVEMENTS: LITTLE FINGER STRIKE

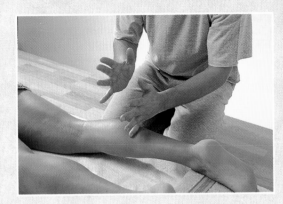
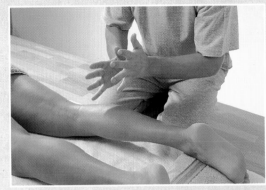

1 Hold the hands above the muscles to be worked on, with the palms facing each other and the fingers apart. Bend each hand sideways from the wrist to strike the tissues with the little finger. In some areas no weight other than that of the hand itself is required; developed muscles may require some added weight. Ensure that the outside border of the palm of the hand does not strike the recipient karate-style.

2 Lift up the striking hand as the second hand comes down to percuss, keeping the hands very close to each other. The hands should rebound from the muscle - be careful not to hit it with a thud. Continue with this alternating striking of the muscles at a slow pace for a few minutes. Work on the length of the muscle group.

When a muscle is subjected to repeated percussive strokes it reacts with minute contractions. If this is kept up for a number of minutes it has a general toning-up effect on the muscle. The technique is best suited to large muscle groups like those of the leg. Care should be taken to avoid delicate areas like the back of the knee.
Note: *To give you some idea of the heaviness required of the little finger strike, imagine you are trying to crack a boiled egg with your little finger. This is the lightest weight required; it can be increased if the muscles are well developed.*

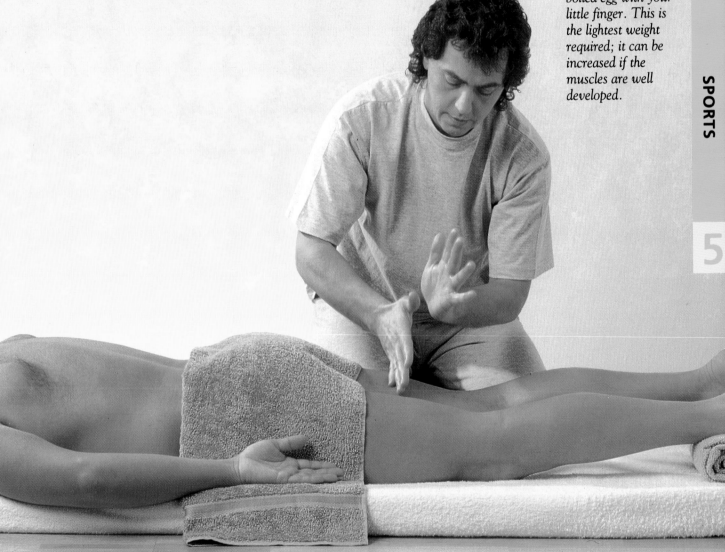

5

PERCUSSIVE MOVEMENTS:CUPPING

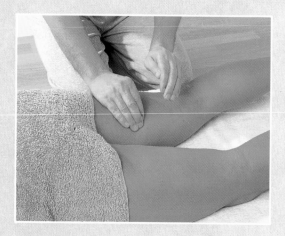

Cupping increases the blood supply and tone of the muscles and the skin. As part of the warm-up routine it can be applied almost anywhere, especially on the leg muscles. Take care to avoid the back of the knee.

1 Place the hands just above the muscle. Cup each hand by curving the palm and fingers, and tighten the whole hand as if you were holding a tennis ball (with the hand held palm-side down and without closing the fingers). The cupped hand strikes the muscle (making a deep sound) as the arm bends from the elbow.

One hand strikes as the other one is lifted off. Let your hands rebound from the muscle rather than hit it with a thud. Continue with this alternating cupping of the tissues for a few minutes and work on the whole area of muscles.

PERCUSSIVE MOVEMENTS: FLAT FIST POUNDING

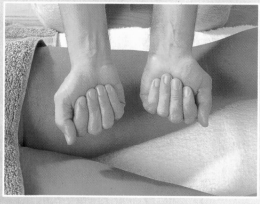

This technique can be used instead of the little finger strike if a heavier weight is required: for example, for bigger muscles.

1 Make a fist but keep the fingers loose and let the tips rest on the heel of the hand. Do not curl them under.

2 Gently strike the muscle tissue with the flat fist, alternating with each hand. Use only the fingers and heel of the hand so the knuckles are not digging into the muscle in any way. Repeat several times along the whole length of the muscle group.

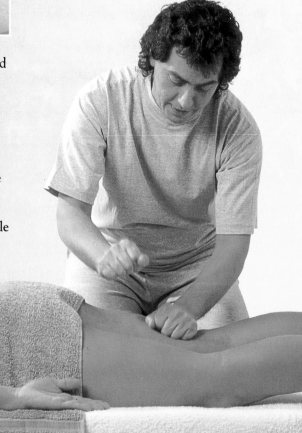

MASSAGE FOR WARMING UP THE BACK

· ·

The back muscles can be warmed by effleurage and percussive strokes. Take care not to let the tissues get chilled before, during or after any warm-up techniques, particularly to the back. Techniques used for warming up include the following strokes.

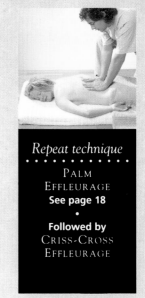

Repeat technique
· · · · · · · · · ·
PALM
EFFLEURAGE
See page 18
•
Followed by
CRISS-CROSS
EFFLEURAGE

· ·

PERCUSSIVE MOVEMENTS: LITTLE FINGER STRIKE

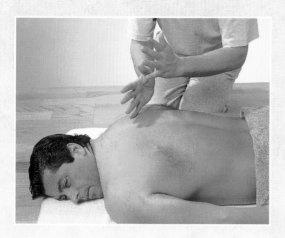

1 *This technique follows palm effleurage and criss-cross effleurage.* The technique with the little fingers (depicted on the leg on page 87) is applied again on the back. It is done to specific muscles only, and areas like the kidneys and the spine should be avoided. The easiest muscles to work on are those on the top of the shoulder, in between the spine and the shoulder blade and on each side of the spine. The percussive strokes are carried out with hardly any weight added to that of the hand itself. If the recipient agrees, the muscles of the buttocks can also be toned up with this technique.

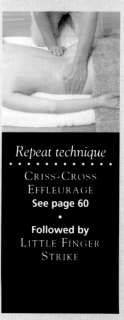

Repeat technique
· · · · · · · · · ·
CRISS-CROSS
EFFLEURAGE
See page 60
•
Followed by
LITTLE FINGER
STRIKE

SPORTS

5

· ·

PERCUSSIVE MOVEMENTS: CUPPING

1 Cupping is also employed to warm up the back. It is used all over the back except over areas like the kidneys and the spine. The muscles and skin tissue of the buttocks also benefit from this movement if the recipient agrees.

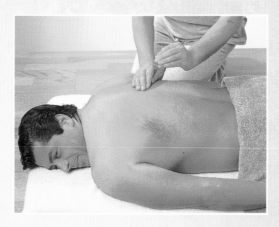

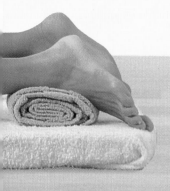

MASSAGE FOR WARMING UP – THE ARM

· ·

The following techniques are used to warm up and tone up the arm muscles. The movements are carried out fairly briskly to increase the temperature. Some require you to be on the opposite side of the recipient's body, so you may want to work on both arms simultaneously.

· ·

PETRISSAGE

Petrissage the arm in the following order:
a) the biceps muscle on the front of the upper arm nearest to you
b) the muscles on the outside of the upper arm furthest away from you.
Then move round to the other side to repeat the procedure.

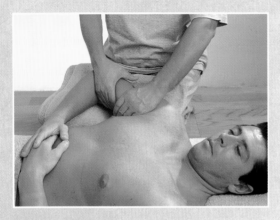

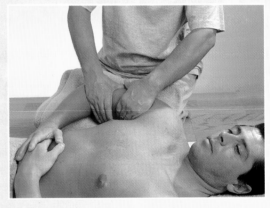

1 *This technique follows effleurage.* To work on the biceps of the arm nearest to you position yourself at the side of the recipient. The arm can rest on a cushion or a folded towel. Lift and gently squeeze the biceps with the fingers of one hand and the thumb of the other (the heel of the hand can be used instead of the thumb). As the fingers and thumb slide towards the centre of the muscle belly ease the compression so as not to pinch the skin.

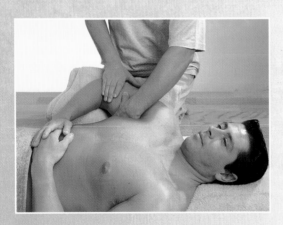

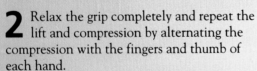

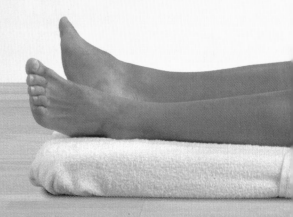

2 Relax the grip completely and repeat the lift and compression by alternating the compression with the fingers and thumb of each hand.

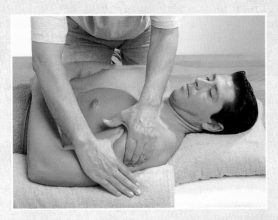

3 The opposite arm can rest on the chest or supported on a folded towel so you can petrissage the triceps and deltoid muscles of the outer and upper arm in the same manner as for the biceps.

Change position and repeat the movements in the same order on the other arm. (Top) compression between fingers of left hand and thumb of right; (middle) compression between fingers of left hand and thumb of right; (bottom) pressure released.

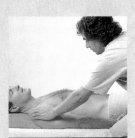

Repeat technique
. . . .
EFFLEURAGE
See page 70
•
Followed by
PETRISSAGE

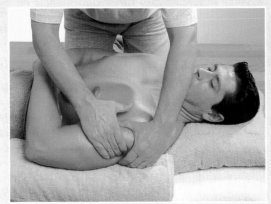

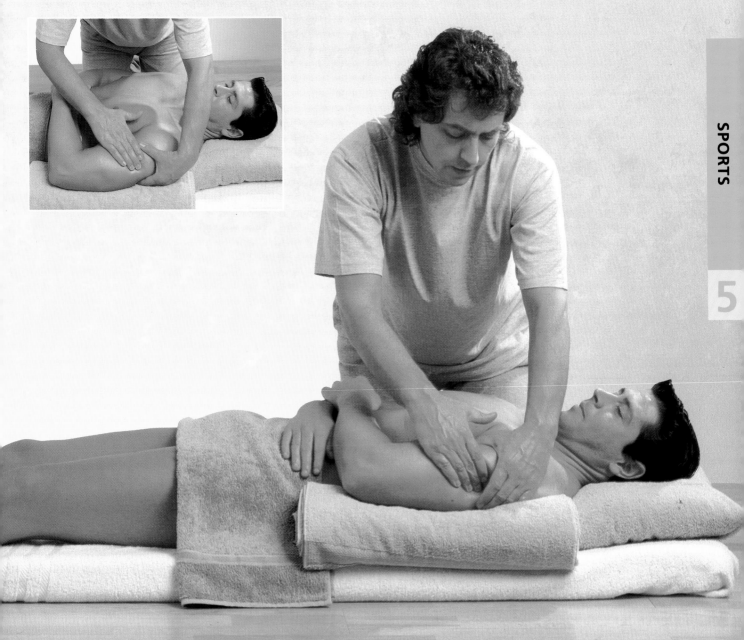

SPORTS

5

PERCUSSIVE STROKES: LITTLE FINGER STRIKE

Carry out the percussive strokes by keeping the hands close together and moving them as one unit to cover the whole muscle group. The little finger strike is carried out with each hand alternately striking the muscle tissue.

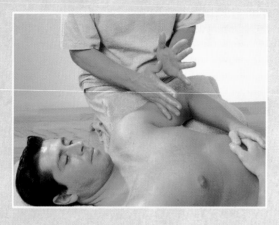

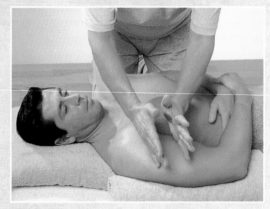

1 Start with the biceps of the arm nearest to you. The little finger strike is done with very little weight and is adapted to the size of these muscles.

2 Adopt the same position as for the previous technique to perform the little finger strike on the outer muscles of the opposite arm.

PERCUSSIVE STROKES: CUPPING

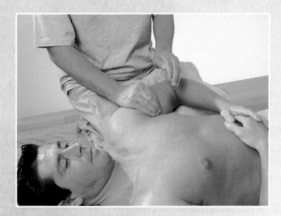

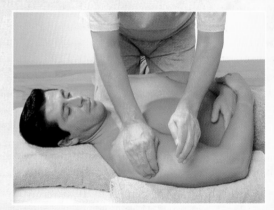

1 Follow the pattern for the previous two movements, working on the biceps of the arm nearest to you first. The cupping movement is done in the same manner as for the back of the legs but the pressure is adjusted according to the size of the muscle.

2 Having completed the movement on the biceps of one arm, reach over to repeat the movement on the triceps of the other.

MASSAGE FOR WARMING UP–
SELF-ADMINISTERED

Anyone participating in sports would benefit from self-administered massage techniques before workouts and sports events. Warming up the muscles reduces the possibility of injury.

PALM EFFLEURAGE – THIGH

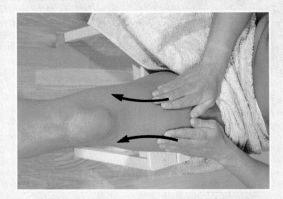

1 Sit on the floor or on a chair and place the hands on the front of one thigh. Effleurage with the palm and fingers down towards the knee, both hands working together.

This effleurage technique is carried out as part of the warm up routine to increase the local circulation.

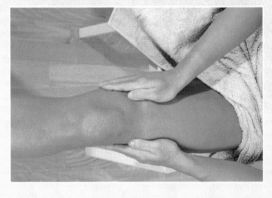

2 Just before the hands reach the knee take one hand to the inside and the other to the outside of the thigh. To complete a circle both hands move up again towards the pelvis. Repeat this briskly several times. Repeat the stroke but with the hands massaging and then travelling up the back of the thigh instead of the outside and inside. Repeat several times.

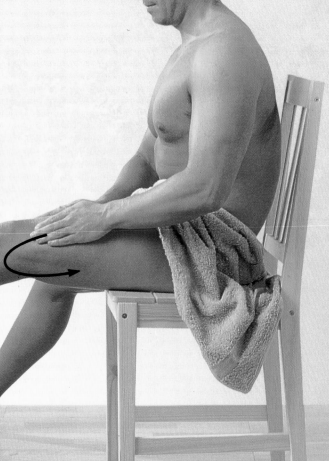

ALTERNATING PALM EFFLEURAGE – CALF

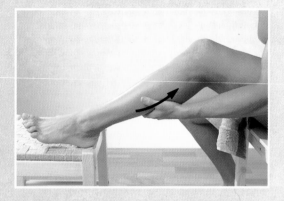 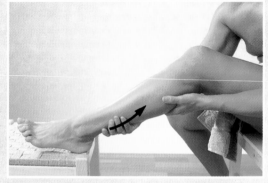

Work on the calf as for the thigh. The stroke is done upwards towards the knee to warm up the tissues and increase circulation.

1 Use the palm and fingers of one hand to effleurage the calf muscle, starting at the lower end and finishing behind the knee. As you work upwards, give a gentle squeeze to the muscles.

2 Follow with the second hand which starts the movement just before the first hand finishes behind the knee. Continue with this alternating stroke in a brisk manner for a few minutes.

CRISS-CROSS EFFLEURAGE – THIGH AND CALF

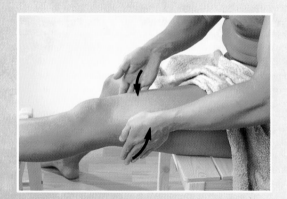 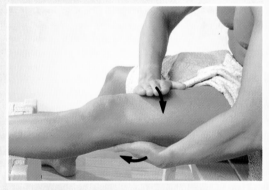

Place the hands on either side of the thigh with your fingers pointing in the same direction, more or less towards the floor. Massage both sides simultaneously (the inside and outside, the front and back). Each hand moves back and forth but in opposite directions, rather like rubbing hands.

1 Place one hand on the inner part of the thigh and the second hand on the outer part. Use a back and forth movement with each hand along the length of the thigh.

2 Place one hand on the front and the second hand on the back of the thigh, with the fingers pointing in opposite directions. Effleurage across the muscle group, travelling along the length of the thigh.

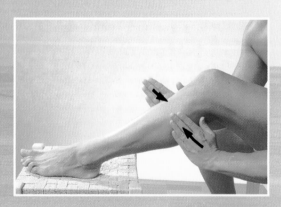

3 Effleurage the calf muscles in the same criss-cross manner. One hand is placed on the inner calf and the second hand on the outer part. The fingers point more or less forwards and the hands move back and forth across the length of the leg. Include as much of the calf muscle as possible, as you work up and down the leg.

MASSAGE FOLLOWING SPORT

Straight after an event like a long run or a cycling tournament the vessels supplying the muscles are engorged. A massage is not necessary at this stage – if it is administered, care must be taken not to apply any heavy pressure. Massage after an event is usually given after one or two hours have elapsed, the object being to reduce any build-up of lactic acid and carbon dioxide. An athlete is likely to have a trained and efficient circulatory system which performs this function so, in theory, massage should not be required. Residual by-products of muscle metabolism tend to linger, however, so a technique to enhance the elimination process is beneficial. Massage oils like camomile and marjoram are used to ease muscular pains and stiffness.

in the area, giving rise to tenderness and pain. Petrissage helps to clear away toxins. It is carried out in conjunction with effleurage and restricted to very tense muscles. The movement is performed using only light pressure. Petrissage techniques for the muscles at the back of the thighs are shown on page 86.

SELF-ADMINISTERED MASSAGE

Palm effleurage is used to improve the circulation and drainage of the legs. Place your hands on either side of the leg. Effleurage from the ankle upwards towards the top of the thigh. Resting the foot on a cushion or on the wall helps with the movement and gravity aids the drainage.

Effleurage after sport

Palm effleurage to the front of the leg (page 72)
•
Palm effleurage to the foot (page 73)
•
Lymph drainage to the lower leg (pages 124 and 127)
•
Lymph drainage to the thigh (page 123)
•
Palm effleurage to the back (page 19)

EFFLEURAGE MOVEMENT

The effleurage movement described previously can be used for post-event massage, with the pressure very much reduced to enhance the drainage of the lymph fluid. Any part of the body will benefit from post-event effleurage, particularly the legs. Opposite are examples of effleurage strokes which can be applied after a sporting event.

PETRISSAGE

A build-up of toxic by-products in the muscles may stimulate the nerve endings

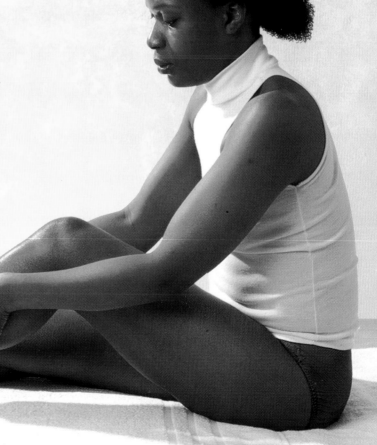

SPORTS

5

SPORTING INJURIES

Most athletes are very keen to tell you about the injuries they have suffered: some will even delight in telling you how brave they were to carry on with their sport despite their injury. Unfortunately, the after-effects of such heroic feats can be excessive scar tissue, impairment of full muscle function and increased susceptibility to further damage. Playing on with an injury is not a requisite for becoming a top athlete. Coming off the field may not be practical for a professional player, but in amateur sports the participant has more of a choice. Whether professional or amateur, the athlete should be able to recognize the injury, stop when necessary and receive the appropriate treatment.

The most common injuries are strains and sprains to muscles, tendons and ligaments. All need proper attention if fur-

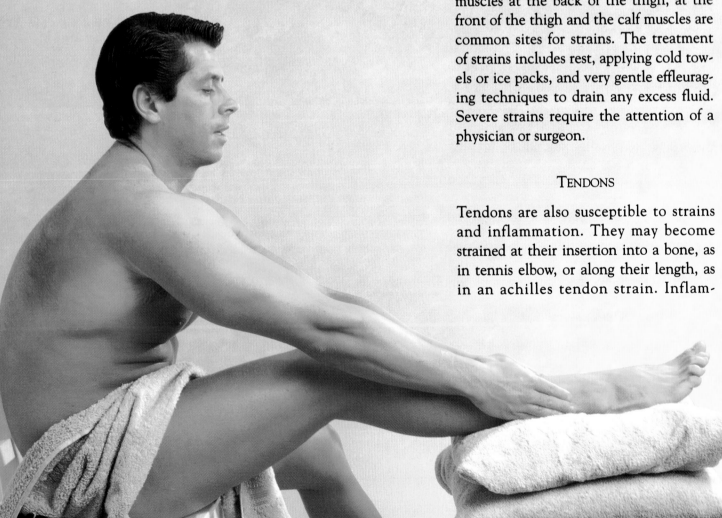

ther damage is to be avoided. Treatment for sporting injuries can vary from one practitioner to another – my theories may differ from those of my colleagues. What matters, however, is that we all achieve the same result. My aim in this book is to offer advice on how to look after an injury if it is a minor one, or until proper treatment is available for more serious problems. This first aid treatment is not a substitute for professional advice.

MUSCLE STRAIN

A strain is a slight tear of the tissue which occurs from over-using, over-stretching or over-loading a muscle. The tear may be in the muscle fibre itself or in the surrounding tissue. In all cases there is some degree of inflammation and a build-up of fluid. Using the muscle causes sharp pain, but at rest it is usually comfortable. The muscles at the back of the thigh, at the front of the thigh and the calf muscles are common sites for strains. The treatment of strains includes rest, applying cold towels or ice packs, and very gentle effleuraging techniques to drain any excess fluid. Severe strains require the attention of a physician or surgeon.

TENDONS

Tendons are also susceptible to strains and inflammation. They may become strained at their insertion into a bone, as in tennis elbow, or along their length, as in an achilles tendon strain. Inflam-

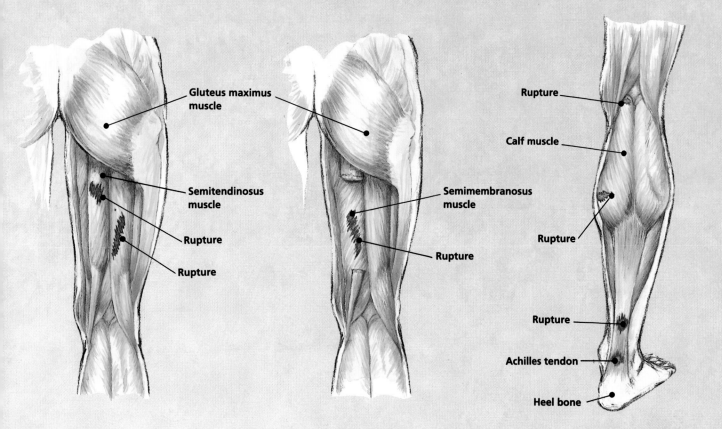

Gluteus maximus
muscle

Semitendinosus
muscle

Rupture

Rupture

Semimembranosus
muscle

Rupture

Rupture

Calf muscle

Rupture

Rupture

Achilles tendon

Heel bone

This diagram shows two very common ruptures of the "hamstrings" group of muscles; the semitendinousus and the biceps femoris.

In this diagram the semitendonus has been cut away to reveal a rupture of the semimembranous muscle, the third muscle of the hamstrings group.

This shows ruptures of one of the calf muscles, the gastrocnemius. The more common areas of injury to this muscle are: at the upper end of the muscle where it joins the femur or thigh bone; at the lower end of the muscle where it joins its tendon; along the tendon itself; where the tendon enters the heel bone.

mation of the tendon (tendinitis) or of its covering sheath (peritendinitis or tenovaginitis) are also common in sports and also in RSI (repetitive strain injury). Pain is experienced on use and the area is very tender to touch. The same procedure of rest, cold packs and gentle draining effleurage applies for tendon strains and inflammation. As with muscles, professional treatment may be needed if the injury is severe.

LIGAMENTS

Ligaments are small bands of non-elastic fibres which hold together the bones which make a joint. They tear if a joint is stretched beyond its normal range of movement. Common sites for this are the outside of the ankle and the inner aspect of the knee. Ligaments have a poorer blood supply than tendons so they can take anything up to twelve weeks to heal. Short of immobilizing the joint in plaster it is difficult to prevent ligaments from being re-stretched and strained again. This also contributes to the prolonged healing period. For the same reason, the fluid which builds up around the joint may take some time to reduce.

As soon as possible after the injury the joint should be immobilized with strapping. Mostly this calls for the expertise of a sports therapist. If the injury is only minor, or as a first aid measure, strapping can be applied safely by the athlete or a helper to prevent further damage. Ice packs or cold towels can also be

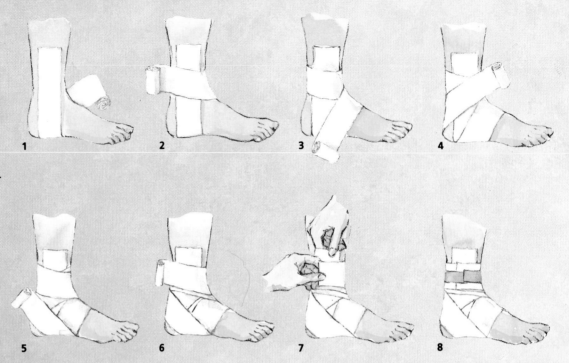

In the case of ligament sprains a 50cm (2in) sticking plaster or non-stretch bandage can be used to strap and support the ankle. Apply the bandage following steps one to eight. Secure the end of the bandage (step 7) with some sticky plaster. Remove the bandage when applying cold packs and seek professional advice if the strain is severe.

applied in conjunction with bandaging for ten minutes before the strapping is fixed in place. The procedure of icing and strapping can be repeated if necessary every few hours. A bowl of water with ice cubes added makes a very convenient ice pack to immerse the foot in.

The only massage technique which does not require expert hands in this situation is effleurage. See the techniques to drain oedema on page 109.

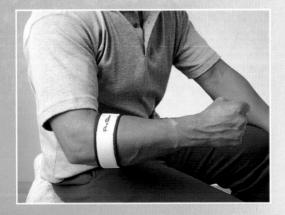

An epicondylitis clip can be used to support the elbow in the case of a tennis elbow injury. Apply the clip, which should have an adjustable tightener, just below the elbow with the hard pad on the outside of the arm. Rest the arm as much as possible and seek professional advice if the injury is severe or chronic.

BURSITIS

Muscles and tendons rub over each other and over bones as they contract and extend during exercise. This would create a lot of friction were it not for tiny little sacs called bursae which have been placed by nature in the most vulnerable areas. Bursae are found between layers of muscles, and between tendons and bones, for example around the knee joint and behind the elbow. Despite the help we get from nature, friction is not completely eliminated in certain situations.

The bursae themselves can become inflamed from over-use. This inflammation is called bursitis, and it used to be very common in the knee due to prolonged periods of kneeling (housemaid's knee) and standing (baker's cyst). But it can also be caused by sports injuries. The elbow joints, and even more commonly the shoulder joints, are also susceptible to this condition. As the onset can be very gradual and the symptoms minimal, it may go unnoticed or, worse still, ignored at first. Recognition of the early signs of bursitis by keeping a watch for heat and inflammation, and then stopping any activity which may be causing it, is the best way of solving the problem. Rest,

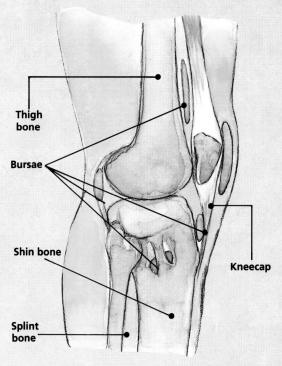

Thigh
bone

Bursae

Shin bone

Splint
bone

Kneecap

together with ice packs or cold towels, are the best form of treatment.

LYMPH DRAINAGE

To reduce oedema (fluid retention) of the leg, the techniques shown on pages 105 and 109 can be applied. This is only a first aid measure, however, and not a substitute for professional treatment.

ICE PACKS

Cooling an area of inflammation will reduce the heat, pain and fluid build-up. Before putting the pack on to the skin apply oil or cream to prevent skin burns. Any small cuts should be covered with plaster to avoid irritation. Apply the ice pack to the area and leave for about ten minutes. Repeat two or three times a day.

Bursae prevent excessive friction between tendons and bones when muscles move the joint. Overuse of muscles can lead to inflammation in one or more of the bursae around the knee joint. The bursa in

front of the kneecap, for example, is apt to become inflamed after extensive kneeling. (see below)

Take care not to:

Apply ice packs if any of the following conditions are present:
Open wounds
•
Excessive bleeding
•
Infections
•
Unexplained heat
•
Cancer
•
Viruses

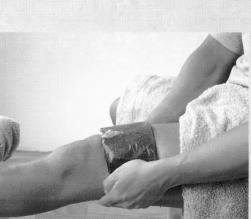

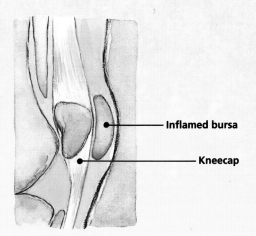

Inflamed bursa

Kneecap

TYPES OF ICE PACK

Commercial ice packs are easily available – some of them are re-useable.

•

A towel which has been immersed in cold water also makes a good ice pack. It has to be refreshed every few minutes to keep it cool, but it is the cheapest treatment and very effective. The water can contain broken ice-cubes to make it colder.

•

Ice broken in small pieces can also be wrapped in a towel as another form of ice pack.

•

The foot can be immersed in a bowl of water to which broken ice-cubes have been added.

SPORTS

5

99

JOINT PAINS

. . . .

To turn each page of this book you have used some twenty joints in the fingers, wrist and elbow. Every movement of the body involves at least one joint. We use our joints constantly and put them under a lot of mechanical stress. The knee, for example, is under about 1.75 kg per sq cm (25 lb per sq in) of pressure during standing. This is about the same pressure a car tyre takes. It is doubled during walking and quadrupled during running.

Most joints are made up of two bones, and there are several different types of joint in the body. A tooth in its socket is one type, called a fixed joint. The main group of joints, and the ones most susceptible to wear and tear, have a membraneous covering called the synovial membrane which forms a capsule round the joint. They are called synovial joints. The end of each bone is covered with a lining called hyaline cartilage which prevents friction between the two bones, assisted by a thick lubricating fluid released by the synovial membrane. As a result of overuse, and as part of the ageing process, the hyaline cartilage can wear out. This leads to complications in various ways, but mostly to pain and inflammation. "Arthritis" means inflammation of a joint. Osteo-arthritis refers to inflammation which is mostly a consequence of wear and tear, and is a frequent development in later life in weight-bearing joints like those of the knee, hip and spine. The familiar "crackling" noises which are commonly audible on movement of the knee joint are due to wear and tear of the under surface of the knee cap, a condition known as chondromalacia patella.

Rheumatoid arthritis refers to a more serious condition which affects not only the cartilage and synovial membrane around the joints but also other tissues of the body. It occurs typically in the smaller joints like those of the hands and feet, but can equally affect larger ones like the knee. Treatment of any form of arthritis requires the attention of a doctor or a complementary practitioner. But you can help reduce some of the inflammation and pain by gentle massage, cold packs and essential oils.

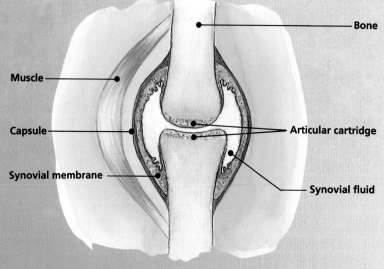

Bone

Muscle

Capsule

Articular cartridge

Synovial membrane

Synovial fluid

This diagram shows the structure of a synovial joint. The synovial membrane lines the inside of the joint ligaments (capsule) and also the part of the bone forming the joint. The articlar (hyaline) cartilage covers the end surfaces of the bones forming the joint and protects the bones as they rub against each other. Tendons cross over the joint which moves as the muscles contract.

PRECAUTIONS

It is not advisable to massage someone when certain conditions are present or certain areas of the body. Instead, seek treatment by a qualified practitioner. Such conditions include the following: Osteoporosis, spondylitis of the cervical spine (neck), cancer of joints, where there is excessive heat in a joint, where there is excessive fluid in a joint.

Wherever there is inflammation there is fluid. Its function is to bring cells to the area to fight off infection and materials to rebuild damaged tissue. Although this is a very efficient process, an excess of fluid can build up as a complication of the condition itself or because the body is overdoing its protective functions. Another factor could be the malfunction of the drainage system taking away the excess fluid. Whatever the reason, excess fluid causes swelling, which increases the pressure within the tissues, which irritates the nerve endings and results in pain.

Cold Compress

Methods to reduce the swelling or oedema are very valuable. One of these is the application of a cold compress. A towel is immersed in a bowl of cold water, wrung out to remove any excess water, and applied to the area for ten to fifteen minutes. As it warms up it can be refreshed by wetting it again. The process is repeated several times during a session. A cold compress is very beneficial during an inflammatory attack when heat is also present, and it can be applied as many times as necessary. If, however, the presence of excess fluid is related to a serious pathological condition, compresses must not be used as a substitute for more intensive treatment.

A few drops of essential oils can be added to the water in which the towel is soaked to enhance its effect. Drop them gently so they float on the surface – and carefully pick them up with the wet towel as you raise it from the bowl. The choice of oils depends on the desired effect – see chart as a guide. Mixing one or two oils can increase the therapeutic value of your application.

Warm Compress

Generally speaking a cold compress has the effect of encouraging fluids away from an area, and a warm compress has the opposite effect, so it is applied to increase the circulation, and thus the heat, to an area like a joint. Osteo-arthritic joints can benefit considerably from an increased blood supply. Improved circulation brings nutrients to the damaged tissues and reduces toxins which could contribute to the condition. Heat in the form of hot baths or compresses is one way of achieving this. The application is similar to that of a cold compress, with the water very warm but not too hot. It is generally

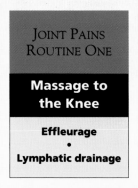

JOINT PAINS ROUTINE ONE
Massage to the Knee
Effleurage · Lymphatic drainage

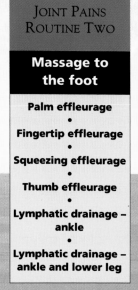

JOINT PAINS ROUTINE TWO
Massage to the foot
Palm effleurage · Fingertip effleurage · Squeezing effleurage · Thumb effleurage · Lymphatic drainage – ankle · Lymphatic drainage – ankle and lower leg

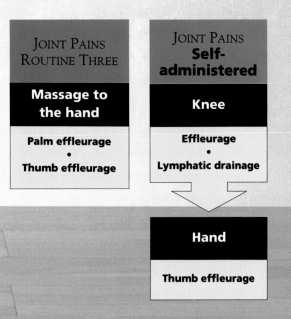

JOINT PAINS ROUTINE THREE
Massage to the hand
Palm effleurage · Thumb effleurage

JOINT PAINS **Self-administered**
Knee
Effleurage · Lymphatic drainage

Hand
Thumb effleurage

6

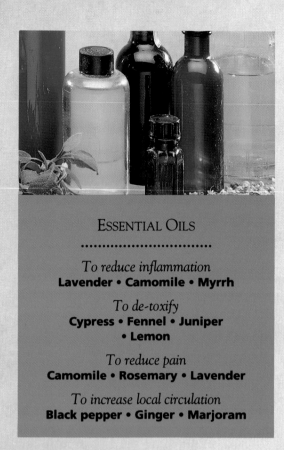

minute. Repeat the process for about ten minutes and always finish with the cold water. As with warm compresses this technique is not used when there is any inflammation or heat present, but it is very beneficial otherwise. Essential oils may be used in the water or rubbed on afterwards.

ESSENTIAL OILS

....

To reduce inflammation
Lavender • Camomile • Myrrh

To de-toxify
**Cypress • Fennel • Juniper
• Lemon**

To reduce pain
Camomile • Rosemary • Lavender

To increase local circulation
Black pepper • Ginger • Marjoram

MASSAGE

Effleurage is perhaps the most appropriate technique for massaging around joints. Very light digital effleurage can be used on some areas, with exceptionally light pressure adjusted according to the feedback from the recipient. It may be best to abandon the massage altogether if even the lightest of pressure causes pain.

safe to apply it a number of times, but warm compresses must not be used on areas of heat or inflammation.

Essential oils can be used in the water in the same way as for a cold compress. Choose an oil for detoxication or for circulation or both – see chart above.

CONTRAST BATHING

Contrast bathing is a very practical way of increasing the circulation to joints in the feet and hands. Two bowls are used, one containing cold, the other very warm, but not hot, water. Submerge the hands or feet in one bowl for a minute, then in the other bowl for another

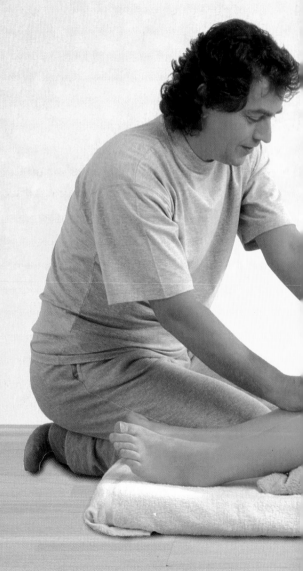

THE KNEE

· ·

The knee joint is very susceptible to pain from arthritic changes, bursitis and so on.
In addition to the hot or cold compresses described earlier, the area will benefit
from the following massage technique.

· ·

EFFLEURAGE –
TO INCREASE CIRCULATION

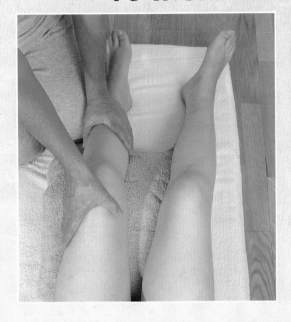
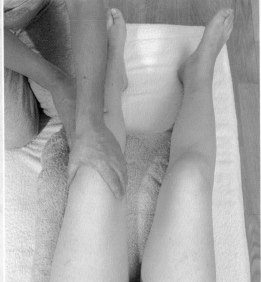

Effleurage the knee to increase the circulation to the joint. This has a very pleasant and warming effect. Use a steady rhythm but not fast. Do not do this technique if excessive pain or heat is present.

1 The recipient lies face upwards. Place a cushion underneath the knee (or under both knees if it is more comfortable). Start with one hand just below the knee, the fingers resting on one side and the thumb on the other side. Effleurage the knee, letting the hand take the shape of the knee itself as you move it towards the lower end of the thigh.

2 Repeat the same stroke with the other hand, starting from just below the knee. Repeat the effleurage several times with both hands, alternating the stroke. Alternatively, repeat the same stroke several times using one hand only.

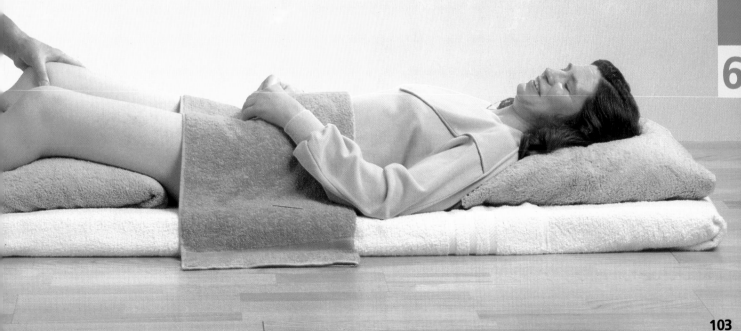

6

SELF-ADMINISTERED EFFLEURAGE – TO INCREASE CIRCULATION

The same effleurage technique can be applied as a self massage. If it is more comfortable, adapt the movement so that one hand is used instead of both.

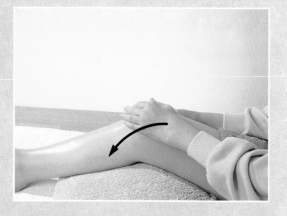

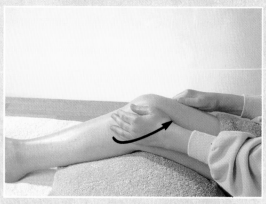

1 The same technique can be applied as a self massage. Sit on the floor or on a chair with one hand placed on top of the thigh just above the knee. The second hand is placed to the side. The upper hand starts the movement by travelling over the knee towards the foot.

2 Once over the knee it moves to the side of the knee and then up again to the thigh to complete a circle.

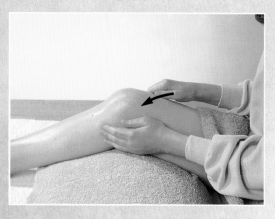

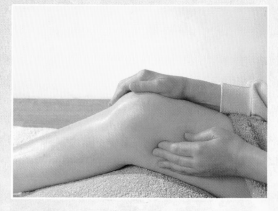

3 The second hand follows the first and moves from the side of the knee to the front of the thigh.

4 From here it travels down over the knee, on to the side and completes a circle as it returns to the front of the thigh. In this fashion the hands follow each other and each hand in turn completes a circle as it effleurages around the knee.

LYMPH DRAINAGE EFFLEURAGE –
TO REDUCE OEDEMA

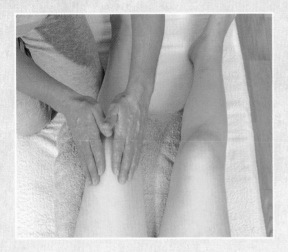

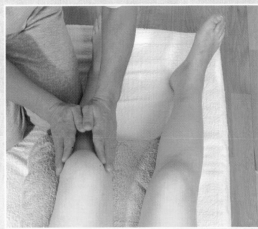

1 Place the flat fingers of each hand next to each other just above the knee. Maintaining a light pressure, effleurage upward toward the top of the thigh. When you get halfway up the thigh, return to the knee and repeat the movement several times. Take about eight seconds to complete each stroke.

2 Place one hand on the inside and the other on the outside of the knee and repeat the effleurage movement. Move as far as the middle of the thigh, lift the hands off gently, and return to the first position. Repeat the stroke several times.

This effleurage is very slow and requires only the weight of the hand with hardly any pressure, almost as if you were feeling the texture of a fine material like velvet. The movement is repeated ten or twenty times to achieve the desired effect of draining the fluid. Several strokes are described here for treating the knee area, each one moving fluid upwards towards the inguinal nodes ("filtering stations" in the groin) at the top of the thigh. To give some idea of the speed – to effleurage from below the knee to the middle of the thigh (as in step 2) takes about six seconds.

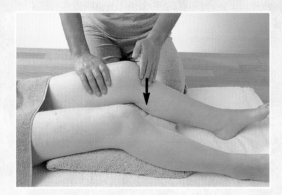

3 Place one hand only across the front part of the knee just below the kneecap, with the fingers pointing towards the inner aspect of the knee. Effleurage with this one hand (a very short, light movement) from the centre towards the back of the knee. This follows the fluid drainage channels in this area. The other hand rests lightly on the thigh but is not used.

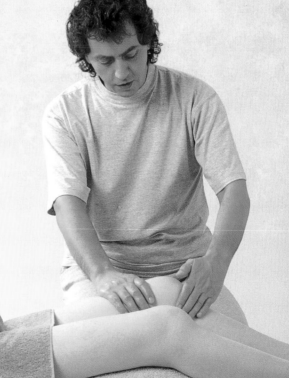

SELF-ADMINISTERED LYMPH DRAINAGE EFFLEURAGE

This is similar to the effleurage for circulation, but carried out with very little pressure. As with the previous effleurage you may want to adapt the movement so that one hand is used instead of both, particularly if you have arthritis of the hands.

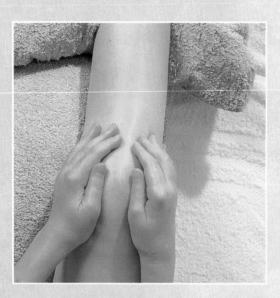

1 To help with the draining of the fluid, raise your leg slightly by placing a cushion underneath it. Effleurage lightly with both hands together, close to each other. Start from below the knee and work upwards until you reach the middle of the thigh.

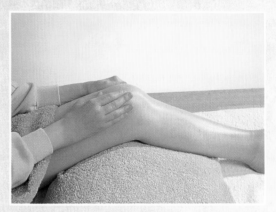

2 Return the hands to below the knee and repeat the movement. Change the position of the hands with each repetition so that the whole area around the knee is covered. Follow the same guidelines on pressure and speed as for administered massage.

THE FOOT

*When massaging the foot take care not to apply too much pressure too quickly.
This is to avoid causing any pain if tender arthritic changes are present.*

Take care not to:
. . . .
Massage the foot if verrucas, athlete's foot or any other contagious skin condition is present.

. . . .

PALM EFFLEURAGE –
TO INCREASE CIRCULATION

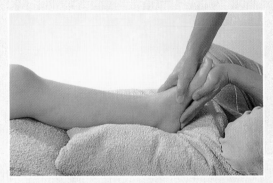 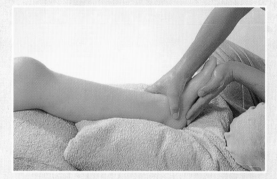

1 The recipient lies face upwards with a cushion under both knees and another one under the foot being massaged. Support the foot with one hand on the sole and the other on the top of the foot.

2 Effleurage the top of the foot from the toes towards the ankle. Apply a little pressure and let the hand follow the shape of the foot. Cover as much of the area as possible with each stroke.

These effleuraging techniques can be used to deal with bad foot circulation. They are useful for most people, particularly when the person is inactive due to illness or some other condition.

. . . .

FINGERTIP EFFLEURAGE –
TO INCREASE CIRCULATION

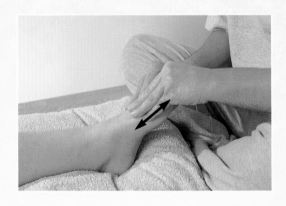 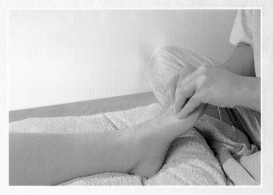

1 Position the fingertips of both hands on the top of the foot with the thumbs underneath. The stroke is done with the fingertips travelling towards the ankle and back again towards the toes. Adjust the pressure according to the bone structure and comfort of the recipient.

2 Move the fingers to a new position along the top of the foot if necessary to cover the whole area.

Another form of effleurage is done by moving the fingertips back and forth over the top of the foot. The stroke is repeated several times before moving the fingers to a new position.

JOINT PAINS

6

SQUEEZING EFFLEURAGE –
TO INCREASE CIRCULATION

This technique is particularly good for increasing circulation towards the toes. Repeat the movement several times at a steady rhythm.

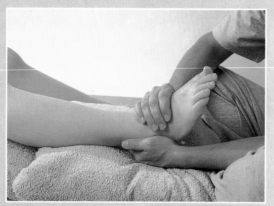 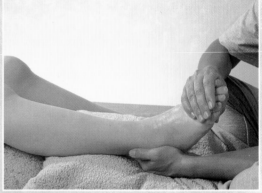

1 With one hand lift and support the foot at the ankle. Place the fingers of the second hand across the top of the foot with the thumb across the sole. Starting at the heel, effleurage towards the toes as you gently squeeze the foot between the fingers and thumb.

2 Go over the toes, reducing the pressure if necessary, and return to the heel end of the foot to repeat the movement.

THUMB EFFLEURAGE – TOES

Handle the toes with care as they can be very tender for some people. In addition to massage, you can try moving the toe to loosen the joints.

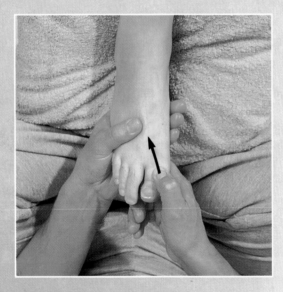 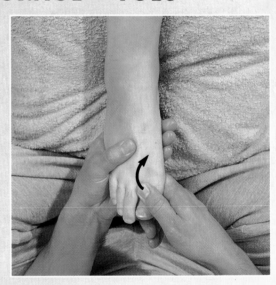

1 The thumb is used to effleurage over the top of each toe while the first finger acts as a support underneath. Movement is with the thumb only, in a circular direction or as a backwards and forwards stroke.

2 Change the position of the thumb if need be so as to cover the whole length of the toe. Repeat several times and treat all the toes.

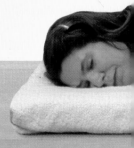

LYMPH DRAINAGE EFFLEURAGE – TO REDUCE OEDEMA OF ANKLE

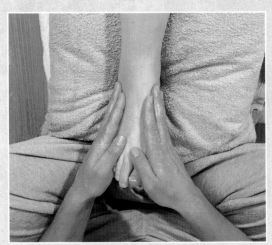 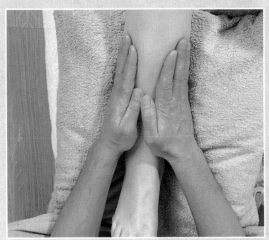

Fluid around the ankle is a sign of bad circulation, or of inflammation, or of both. The lymph drainage massage helps to reduce the oedema but should not be done if excessive heat or pain is present. Cold towels can also be used to reduce fluid and inflammation.

1 The recipient lies face upwards with the foot raised on a cushion. One hand is on the inside and the other on the outside of the ankle.

2 Effleurage lightly over the inside and outside ankle bones, and upwards towards the knee. When you get to halfway along the calf, or to the knee if you can reach comfortably, lift off the hands and return to the first position. Repeat several times.

LYMPH DRAINAGE EFFLEURAGE – LOWER LEG AND ANKLE

This technique can be used in addition to the previous one, or as a substitute.

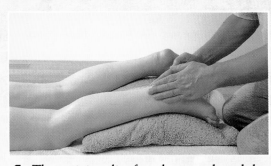

2 When you reach the level of the knee, or just below, return the hands to the first position to repeat the movement.

1 The recipient lies face downwards and the effleurage starts at the ankle and is taken towards the back of the knee. Resting the lower leg on a cushion will help the drainage.

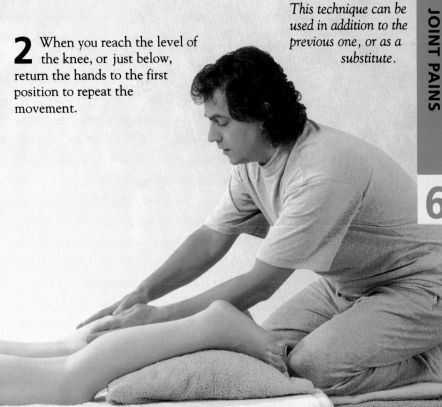

JOINT PAINS

6

THE HAND

· ·

The hands can be very tender to work on, so start the movements gently and
adjust the pressure according to the feedback from the recipient.

· ·

PALM EFFLEURAGE

A recipient who finds lying down difficult may prefer to sit on a chair. The techniques can be easily adapted if the recipient is on the floor.

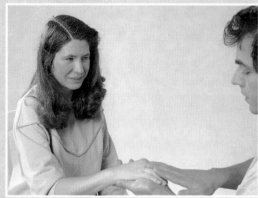

1 The recipient's hand rests on your palm. With your second hand effleurage the back of his or her hand, starting at the fingers and travelling over the wrist. Continue along the lower arm as far as you can reach comfortably. Return the hand to the first position and repeat the movement.

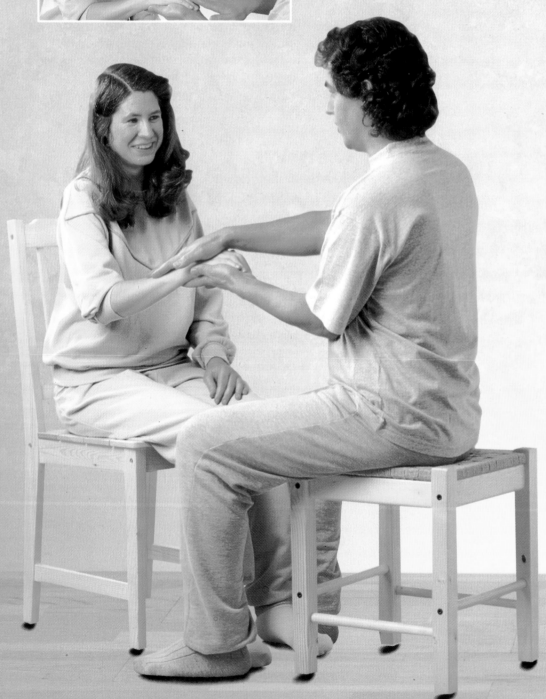

THUMB EFFLEURAGE

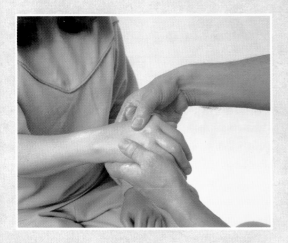

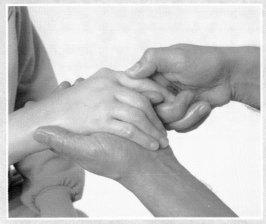

Massage the fingers to increase the circulation. You can also move each finger about to loosen the joints while you are massaging, as long as this is not painful for the recipient.

1 Support the hand while massaging the back of the hand with the thumbs. Move the thumbs in small circles or in a back and forth action. Use the same stroke for the back and front of the wrist.

2 Continue the action down the fingers. Effleurage each finger, using the thumb to carry out the stroke and the first finger as support.

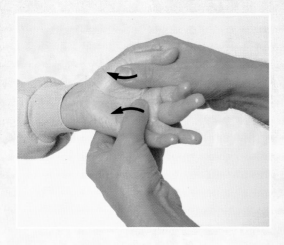

3 In the same manner, both thumbs are used to effleurage the palm of the hand.

SELF-ADMINISTERED THUMB EFFLEURAGE

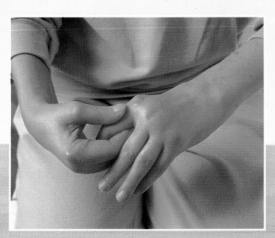

1 Use the thumb of one hand to effleurage the fingers, and the back and palm of the other hand as described above. Adjust the position of the massaging hand, the extent of the stroke and the pressure according to your needs.

Thumb massage can be used on the hand as a self-massage technique. If this is not comfortable for you, use the hand or fingers.

6

CHAPTER 7

PREGNANCY

PREGNANCY

....

Massage in pregnancy has several uses provided it is carried out with care. As the first three months are crucial it is advisable, as a safeguard, not to massage the abdomen during this period, and not to use certain essential oils (see box below). Provided this advice is heeded, there are many benefits of massage during pregnancy.

Submandibular node

Cervical node

Right lymphatic duct

Right subclavian vein

Thymus gland

Lymphatic vessel

Left internal jugular vein

Left subclavian vein

Axillary node

Thoracic duct

Spleen

Small intestine

Intestinal node

Large intestine

Appendix

Iliac node

Inguinal node

Lymphatic vessel

The lymph system is made up of vessels which drain fluid from the skin and superficial tissues and from organs like the small intestines and the spleen. The lymph is filtered as it passes through lymph nodes and eventually drains into two main channels, the right lymphatic duct and the left thoracic duct. These in turn empty into the left and right subclavian veins, thus mixing with blood to be pumped out again by the heart.

The area most likely to need attention is the lower back. As the muscles in this region are used to counterbalance the extra load at the front they are likely to be contracted and tense, giving rise to backache or soreness. Massage helps to reduce the muscle spasm and to lessen any congestion in the tissues.

Massage also provides a pleasant way of keeping the skin moisturized and soft. Some of the essential oils, as well as most

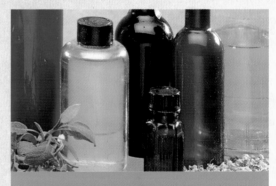

MASSAGE OILS FOR PREGNANCY

....

Use in moderation during pregnancy
**Camomile • Lavender • Lemon •
• Lemongrass • Petitgrain**

Used to prevent stretch marks
Neroli • Mandarin

*The following oils **must not** be used during the first 3-4 months of pregnancy.*
**Aniseed • Armoise (mugwort)
• Arnica • Basil • Clary sage
• Cypress • Fennel • Geranium
• Hyssop • Jasmine • Juniper
• Marjoram • Melissa • Myrrh
• Origanum • Pennyroyal
• Peppermint • Rose • Rosemary
• Sage • Thyme • Wintergreen**

of the commercially available creams, can be used safely for this purpose. Circulation to the legs may be impaired during pregnancy due to the compression of some of the pelvic blood vessels. Massage techniques help to increase the circulation and can be given with the recipient lying comfortably on her back or side. The relaxing and supportive benefits of massage can be enjoyed throughout the pregnancy and, in some cases, right up to labour.

Some of the massage techniques demonstrated in this section use a massage couch or plinth. A large table may also be used, but the movements can be just as easily carried out on the floor. The recipient will probably be most comfortable lying on her side with cushion support if necessary. Some techniques are demonstrated with the recipient sitting on a stool.

MASSAGE OILS

During pregnancy there are more essences which must not be used than there are safe ones. Some essential oils can be slightly toxic; others are described as "emmenagogue", which means that they tend to bring on menstruation and so they are avoided to guard against any chance of miscarriage. Some oils can be used in moderation, like camomile and lavender, but these too are emmenagogue so they should not be used in the early months if there is the slightest chance of a miscarriage. Although the list of oils which should not be used is quite long, some of the citrus oils like lemon, lemongrass and mandarin can still be used. To avoid any risk, massage during the early stages of pregnancy can be done with a vegetable oil such as almond.

DURING PREGNANCY ROUTINE ONE

Massage to the back/Side lying

Palm effleurage
•
Thumb effleurage
•
Lymph drainage

Massage to the back/Sitting

Palm effleurage
•
Heel of hand effleurage
•
Thumb effleurage
•
Lymph drainage

Massage to the abdomen

Palm effleurage
•
Lymph drainage

Massage to the legs

Palm effleurage
•
Lymph drainage

FOLLOWING CHILDBIRTH ROUTINE TWO

Massage to the front of the leg

Palm effleurage
•
Criss-cross effleurage
•
Petrissage
•
Percussive movements
•
Lymph drainage – thigh
•
Lymph drainage – knee
•
Lymph drainage – ankle

Massage to the back of the leg

Palm effleurage
•
Criss-cross effleurage
•
Petrissage
•
Percussive movements
•
Lymph drainage – thigh
•
Lymph drainage – ankle

Massage to the loin area

Palm effleurage
•
Criss-cross effleurage
•
Petrissage
•
Percussive movements
•
Lymph drainage

Massage to the abdomen

Palm effleurage
•
Petrissage
•
Lymph drainage

SELF-ADMINISTERED ROUTINE

Pregnancy

Abdomen
•
Effleurage

Following birth

Abdomen
•
Petrissage
•
Thigh petrissage
•
Percussive strokes

BACK

The back is probably the area needing massage most during pregnancy to reduce muscle tightness and improve circulation. Ensure that the back is flat and not curved in while you are carrying out these techniques.

PALM EFFLEURAGE

Effleurage is used for general relaxation, to improve circulation and to ease muscle tightness. In these techniques, as for all others, take care to adjust the pressure according to the feedback from the recipient. The rhythm is fairly slow.

1 Effleurage the uppermost side of the back with fairly light pressure to start with, increased with each stroke.

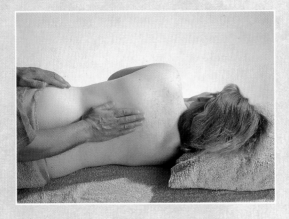

2 The stroke starts at the base of the spine and finishes at the upper back or shoulder. When the treatment is completed, help the recipient to turn on to her other side and carry out the same procedure.

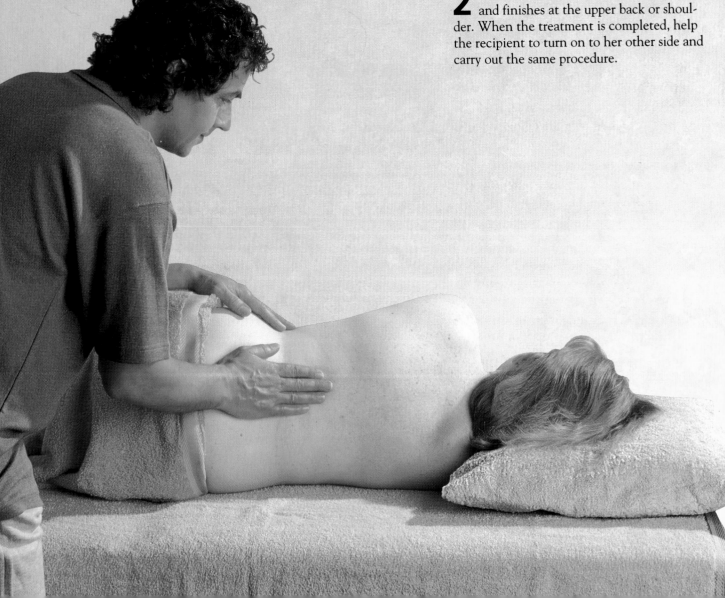

THUMB EFFLEURAGE

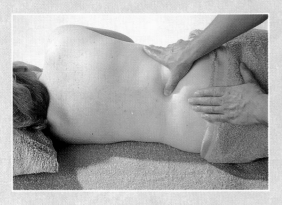

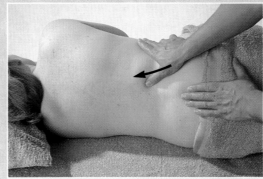

Following the palm effleurage you can work on any tight muscles with the thumb effleurage. Pay particular attention to the muscles of the lower back.

1 In the same position as palm effleurage, apply thumb effleurage to the muscles on the uppermost side running beside the spine. Only one hand is used. The thumb applies most of the pressure as it moves along for about 50cm (2ins).

2 Work on one area with a series of thumb strokes until you feel the muscle softening, then move the hand to a new position and repeat. Work all along the back as far as is comfortable.

LYMPH DRAINAGE EFFLEURAGE

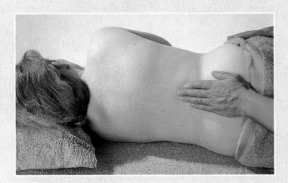

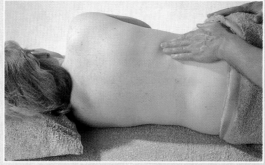

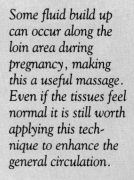

Some fluid build up can occur along the loin area during pregnancy, making this a useful massage. Even if the tissues feel normal it is still worth applying this technique to enhance the general circulation.

1 Draining of any fluid build-up in the lower back is done using this very light effleurage. One or both hands may be used. Start from the centre of the lower back.

2 Effleurage very slowly and lightly along the pelvic bones and over the side of the trunk towards the inguinal nodes (groin area).

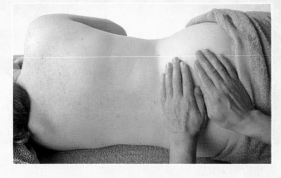

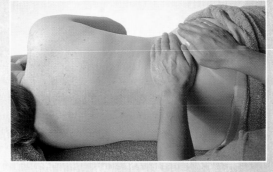

3 It may be more comfortable to use two hands if you are working on a massage plinth or table. If you are working on the floor you may find the single-handed effleurage is easier to perform.

4 Repeat the movement several times, each time working towards the inguinal nodes.

PALM EFFLEURAGE

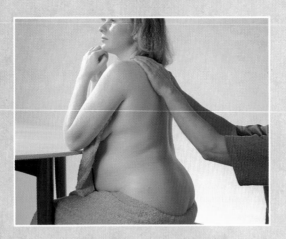 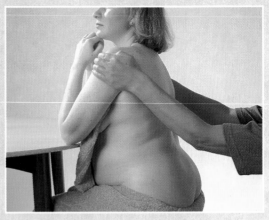

In this sitting position the back can be effleuraged with both hands working from the base of the spine up to and including the shoulders.

1 This is a very soothing and warming-up stroke which can be repeated a number of times. Place the hands on each side of the spine on the lower back with the fingers pointing towards the head (see below). Apply gentle pressure. Effleurage upwards towards the head maintaining an even pressure.

2 Travel to the top of the back, shoulders and upper arm before moving down the outside of the trunk and back to the first position to repeat the stroke.

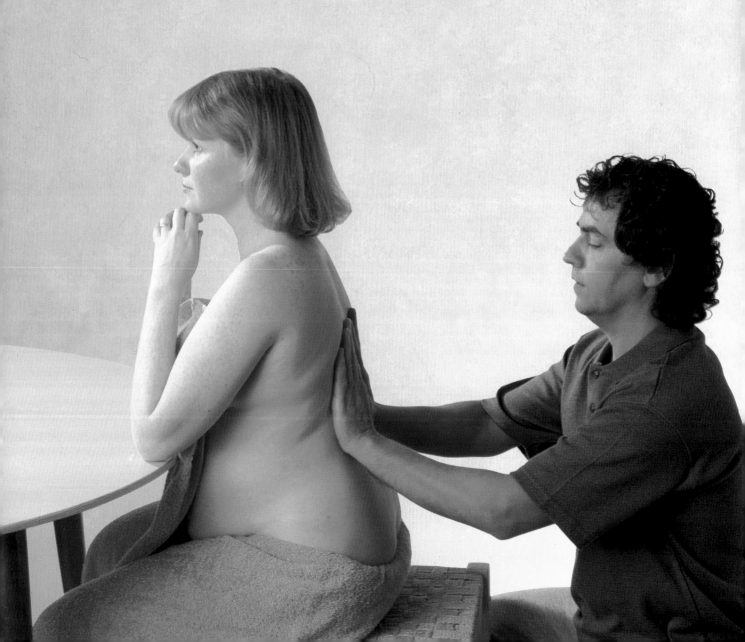

HEEL OF HAND EFFLEURAGE

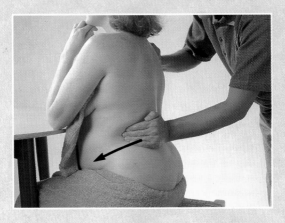

1 Heel of hand effleurage is carried out beside the spine on the side furthest away from you, therefore position yourself to the side of the recipient. Apply pressure with the heel of the hand as you travel across the muscle fibres towards the side of the trunk. The stroke is only a short one, with most of the pressure on the muscle group alongside the spine. Ease off the pressure if you go over the kidney area.

To work more deeply into the muscles, especially those of the lower back which tend to be quite tense, use either heel of hand effleurage or thumb effleurage.

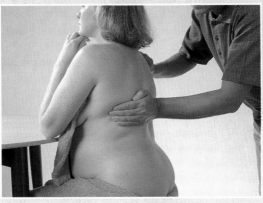

2 Although the lower back is perhaps most suited to this stroke, you can apply it all the way up the side of the spine.

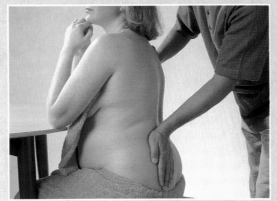

3 Point the fingers towards the floor to carry out the heel of hand effleurage downwards. This is a very good method for relaxing the lower back muscles. Work on both sides of the spine simultaneously.

THUMB EFFLEURAGE

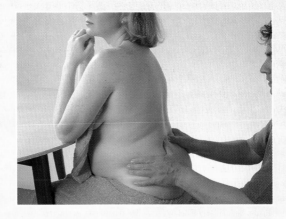

1 Kneel on the floor to position the hands on each side of the back with the thumbs very near the spine. Apply the pressure with the thumbs. Start as far down as you can comfortably reach.

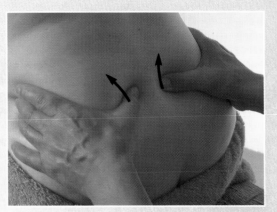

2 Each thumb slides a few inches as the pressure is applied, and the stroke is repeated over the same area a few times. The same stroke is then applied further up the back. Continue the movement as far up the back as you can comfortably reach.

As with heel of the hand effleurage, the thumbs can be used to work more deeply into the muscles.

LYMPH DRAINAGE

Lymph in the lower back drains in two directions and the effleurage we use to help with this drainage follows the same paths. The first one is from the centre of the spine towards the side of the trunk and into the inguinal nodes (groin area). The rest of the fluid drains upwards towards the shoulder and into the armpit. As with all other lymph drainage massage movements, the pressure is extremely light and the movement very slow.

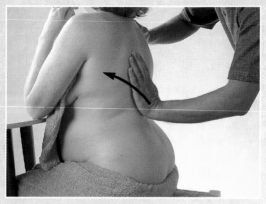

1 For drainage in the inguinal nodes stand or sit on a chair at the side of the recipient and effleurage lightly from the centre of the spine towards the outer trunk on the opposite side with the hand pointing in the same direction or towards the head (see below). Start again with the hand further down towards the buttock to repeat the movement so that the whole area is treated. It takes quite a while for lymph fluid to move along so these strokes are always repeated many times. Stand or sit on the opposite side of the recipient to work on the other side.

2 To help drainage into the axillary (armpit) nodes, effleurage upwards beside the spine and towards the armpit, still working on the side of the spine furthest from you. It is not necessary for the hand to go right under the armpit, but it can do, especially if the recipient has her arms resting on a table.

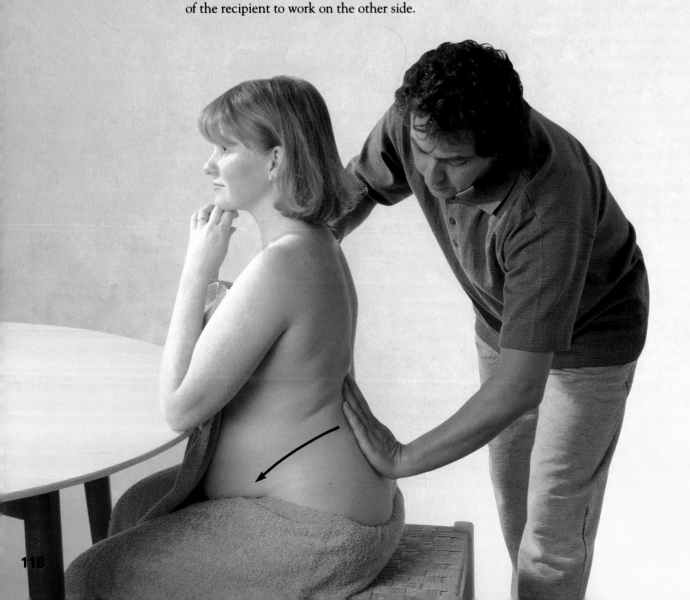

THE LEGS

REPEAT TECHNIQUES

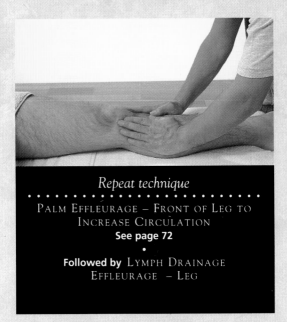

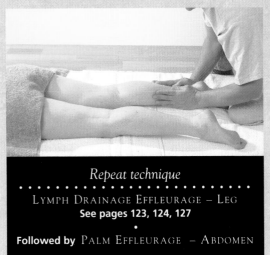

Repeat technique
- - - - - - - - - - - - - - - - - - -
PALM EFFLEURAGE – FRONT OF LEG TO
INCREASE CIRCULATION
See page 72
•
Followed by LYMPH DRAINAGE
EFFLEURAGE – LEG

Repeat technique
- - - - - - - - - - - - - - - - - - -
LYMPH DRAINAGE EFFLEURAGE – LEG
See pages 123, 124, 127
•
Followed by PALM EFFLEURAGE – ABDOMEN

THE ABDOMEN

The recipient lies face upwards.

PALM EFFLEURAGE

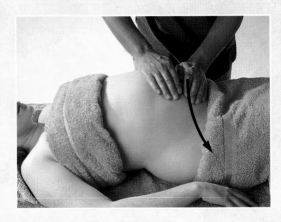

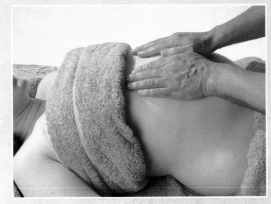

1 Stand beside the recipient with both hands placed next to each other in the centre of her abdomen. Effleurage from the navel towards the inguinal nodes on the opposite side using gentle, not heavy, pressure. When this movement is used for lymph drainage the pressure is reduced to that of the weight of the hand only.

2 Place the hands next to each other in the centre of the abdomen pointing towards the chest. Keeping contact with the palm and fingers, effleurage upwards to the chest or breastbone. Follow the same guide on pressure as in the previous stroke.

Moisturizing creams and oils can be rubbed into the skin using palm effleurage. Fluid can also be drained away with this technique, though this is perhaps more necessary in the post-pregnancy period. The effleurage is done very lightly and follows the two directions of the lymph flow: from the navel down towards the inguinal nodes and from the navel upwards towards the chest.

PREGNANCY

7

SELF-ADMINISTERED EFFLEURAGE

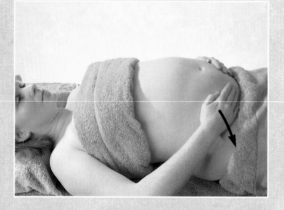 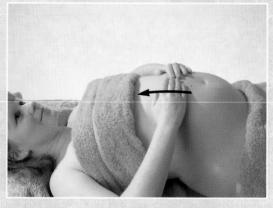

Lying on your back is perhaps the easiest way to apply the same palm effleurage on yourself. Use this stroke to rub in creams and oils.

1 The fingers point towards the middle and the stroke starts at the navel. Following the same guidelines for pressure and application as for the administered massage, effleurage from the navel to the inguinal nodes. In this instance, however, the hands start in the middle but separate so that the right hand moves towards the right groin area and the left toward the left groin area.

2 With the hands back at the navel and the fingers pointing towards each other, effleurage upwards to the chest or breastbone. This is a fairly short stroke but effective when repeated several times.

FOLLOWING CHILDBIRTH

Following childbirth, massage has a very significant function. Given regularly it is beneficial in improving circulation, reducing fluid retention and toning up the muscles and skin.

MASSAGE OILS AFTER CHILDBIRTH

Toning muscles and skin
Black pepper • Juniper • Rosemary

Reducing oedema
Geranium • Rosemary

To help the circulation
Lemon • Camomile • Cypress • Black pepper • Juniper • Marjoram

Skin
Neroli • Frankincense

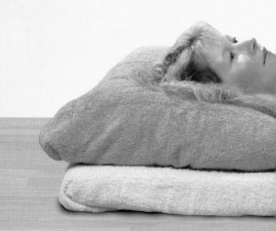

THE FRONT OF THE LEG

The following techniques should be used regularly, perhaps even on a daily basis. Start with very little pressure in all techniques during the first week or so following childbirth and increase this gradually over the following weeks.

CRISS-CROSS EFFLEURAGE – THIGH

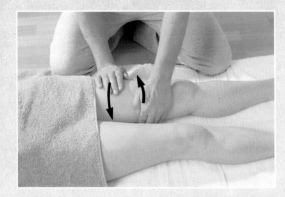

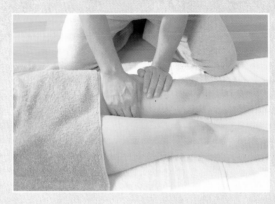

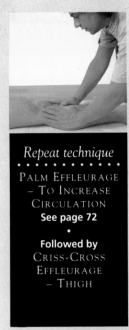

Repeat technique

PALM EFFLEURAGE
– TO INCREASE
CIRCULATION
See page 72
•
Followed by
CRISS-CROSS
EFFLEURAGE
– THIGH

1 *This technique follows palm effleurage.* Position yourself to the side of the recipient. Place both hands on the thigh, one on the outer and one on the inner side with fingers pointing away from you.

2 The hands move across the muscles, towards and past each other (i.e. they alternately travel to the inside and outside of the thigh). Repeat this criss-cross effleurage along the length of the whole thigh.

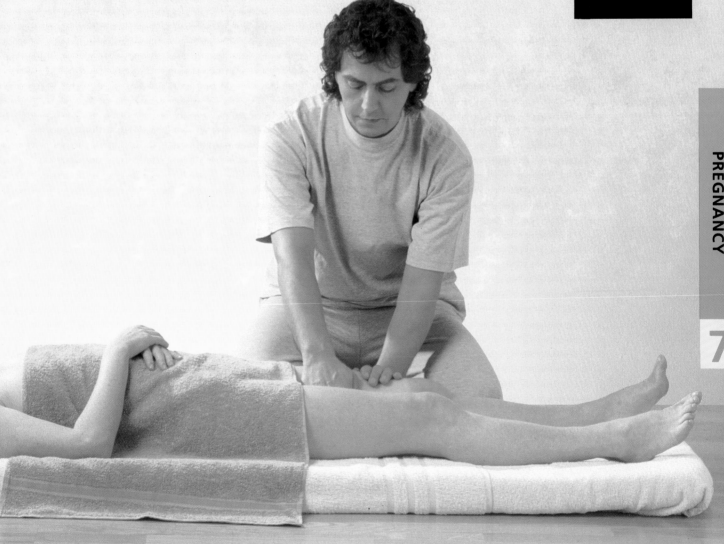

PREGNANCY

7

PETRISSAGE – THIGH MUSCLES

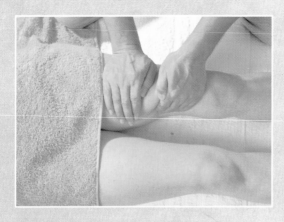

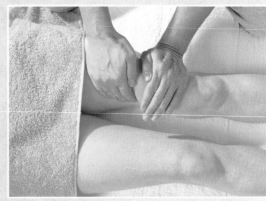

Petrissage lifts the muscle group away from the underlying bone while compressing the muscle tissue. You can use the thumb instead of the heel of the hand.

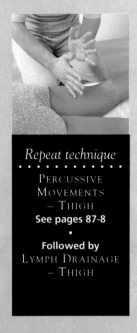

Repeat technique

PERCUSSIVE
MOVEMENTS
– THIGH
See pages 87-8
•
Followed by
LYMPH DRAINAGE
– THIGH

1 Start with the fingers of one hand on the inside of the thigh and the heel of the second hand on the outside. Apply pressure with both hands to compress and lift up the muscle. Add a gentle twist of the tissues at the same time. Continue with the compression but let the hands slide towards each other in the centre. Be careful not to pinch the skin. Reduce the grip and ease the muscle tissue from between your hands.

2 Repeat the movement with the fingers of each hand alternately starting on the inside of the thigh, and the heel of the other hand on the outside. Cover the whole length of the thigh.

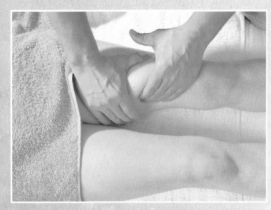

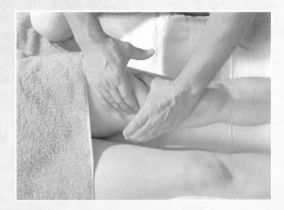

1 Alternatively, the same compressing movement can be carried out between the thumb of one hand against the fingers of the second hand.

2 Petrissage the whole thigh area by applying the compression alternately between the fingers and thumb of each.

LYMPH DRAINAGE – THIGH

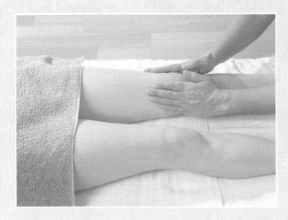

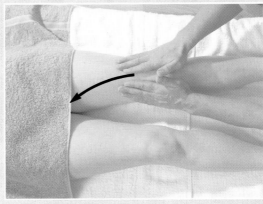

1 *This technique follows percussive movements to the thigh.* The thigh is drained by effleuraging first the outer and then the inner areas. The hands work very close together with contact across the whole hand. From the outer region move very slowly towards the inguinal nodes, taking about eight seconds to travel from the lower to the upper end of the thigh. When you reach the groin area return to the starting position to repeat the movement.

2 Repeat the movement several more times with the hands starting at the inner aspect of the thigh. Effleurage towards the groin area as in the previous stroke.

The flow of lymphatic fluid in the leg is from the ankle to the lymphatic nodes behind the knee and then on to the next group of nodes in the inguinal (groin) area. The effleurage which is used to assist this drainage is first carried out on the thigh to clear the exit pathways of the fluid. This is followed by drainage of the knee and lower leg. Draining requires very light, very slow effleurage, repeated many times.
Note: An excess of local or systemic fluid may require the attention of a general practitioner or a complementary therapist.

LYMPH DRAINAGE – KNEE

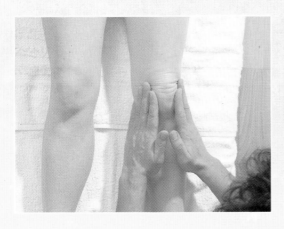

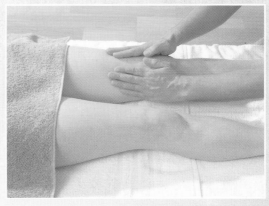

1 Place one hand on the inside and the other on the outside of the knee. Effleurage lightly, as in the previous movement, towards the top of the thigh.

2 Continue the movement as far as the middle of the thigh. Lift off the hands gently and return to the first position for the stroke to be repeated.

Make contact with the palm and the fingers of both hands. Keep the hands relaxed, letting each hand mould itself over the knee as it travels across upwards.

LYMPH DRAINAGE –
LOWER LEG AND ANKLE

As in the other lymphatic drainage movements, the pressure is very light. The feeling as you effleurage toward the knee should be of dragging the hands rather than applying actual pressure. Using a cushion aids drainage, but is not essential.

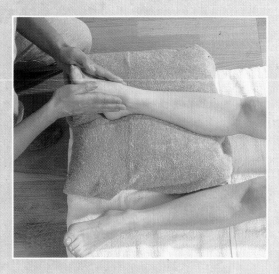

1 The recipient lies on her back with the foot raised on a cushion. Place one hand on the inside and the other on the outside of the ankle, and effleurage from the ankle up towards the knee.

2 Just before you get to the knee both hands travel towards the inside of the leg to finish the stroke. Lift off the hands and return to the first position. Repeat several times.

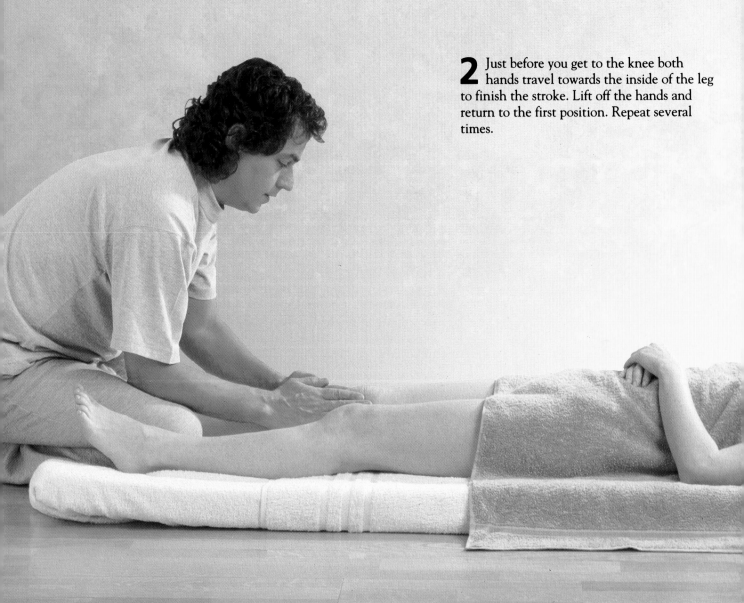

THE BACK OF THE LEG

Massage the back of the legs with the recipient lying face down and, if necessary, using cushions for support under the abdomen, chest and feet.

PALM EFFLEURAGE –
TO INCREASE CIRCULATION

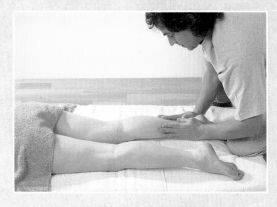

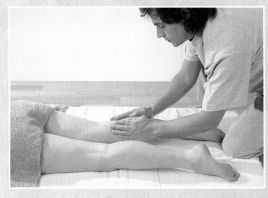

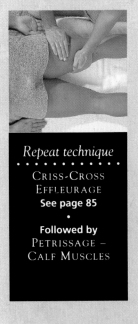

1 This stroke is one complete movement from the ankle to the top of the thigh. Effleurage upwards with the hands next to each other and curved slightly around the leg. Add a little pressure to the movement and a gentle squeeze of the tissues with both hands.

2 Reduce the pressure and lift the hands off a little as you go over the back of the knee.

Repeat technique

CRISS-CROSS
EFFLEURAGE
See page 85

•

Followed by
PETRISSAGE –
CALF MUSCLES

3 As the hands reach the top of the thigh they separate, one travelling to the outside and the other to the inside. With the pressure taken off completely slide the hands down the leg to the ankle so the movement can be repeated.

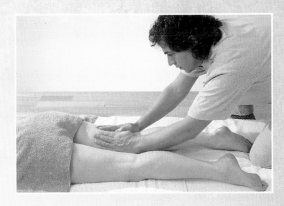

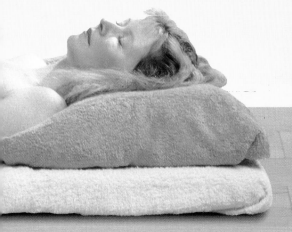

PREGNANCY

7

PETRISSAGE – CALF MUSCLES

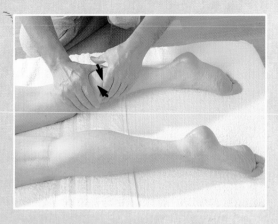

This is carried out in the same manner as for the back of the thigh muscles (see page 86) except that the thumb is used more than the heel of the hand.

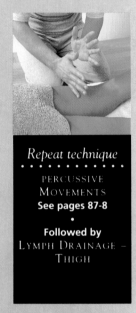

Repeat technique

PERCUSSIVE
MOVEMENTS
See pages 87-8

•

Followed by
LYMPH DRAINAGE –
THIGH

1 *This technique follows criss-cross effleurage (p.125).* Start with the fingers of one hand on the inside of the calf and the thumb of the second hand on the outside (the heel of the hand can be used instead of the thumb). Apply pressure with both hands and begin to compress and lift up the muscle. Add a gentle twist of the tissues at the same time.

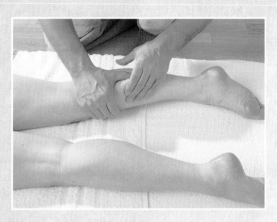

2 Continue with the compression, letting the hands slide towards each other in the centre. Be careful not to pinch the skin. Reduce the grip and ease the muscle tissue from between your hands.

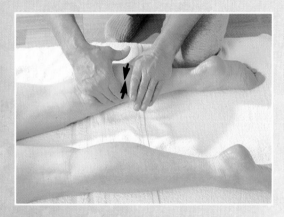

3 Repeat the movement with the fingers of each hand alternately starting on the inside of the calf, and the thumb of the other hand on the outside. Cover the whole length of the calf.

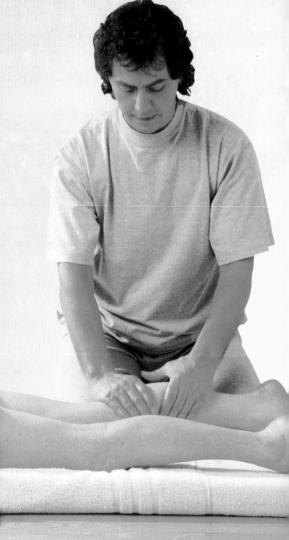

LYMPH DRAINAGE – THIGH

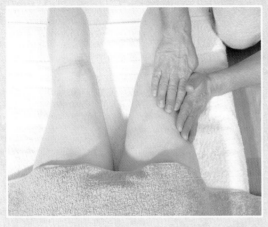

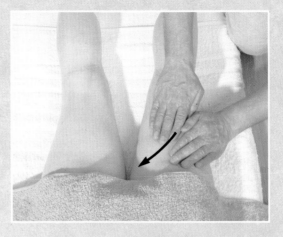

When working on the back of the legs avoid any heavy work on varicose veins or, if they are really bad, omit the massage altogether.

1 *This technique follows percussive movements.* Effleurage with the movement starting on the outer region and from the lower end of the thigh just above the knee. Move the hands close together upwards and across the thigh towards the inner area and the inguinal nodes.

2 Having crossed the thigh, the stroke finishes with the hands very near, but not quite on, the inside of thigh. Repeat the movement several times. Change the position of the hands, if necessary, to cover the whole thigh area.

LYMPH DRAINAGE – LOWER LEG AND ANKLE

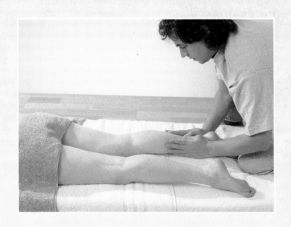

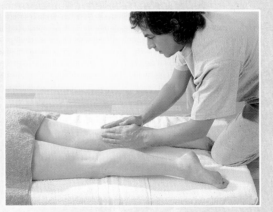

Use this technique in addition to the lymph drainage that was carried out while the recipient was on her back.

1 Resting the lower leg on a cushion will help the drainage. The hands are placed one on the inside and one on the outside of the ankle. Effleurage from the ankle towards the back of the knee.

2 At the knee level or just below it, return the hands to the first position to repeat the movement several times.

THE LOIN AREA

To massage the lower back with the recipient lying face down, it may be necessary to place a pillow or cushion beneath the abdomen, especially following childbirth.

PETRISSAGE

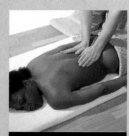

Repeat technique

PALM EFFLEURAGE
– TO LOWER BACK
FOR INCREASING
CIRCULATION
See page 33
•
Followed by
CRISS-CROSS
EFFLEURAGE
– TO LOIN AREA

The loin muscles are situated between the lower ribs and the upper part of the pelvic bone, the iliac crest. These muscles also extend from the front of the abdomen to the spine. This region tends to have a prominent layer or two of fat! Petrissage to this area is therefore very useful not only to increase the local circulation but also for its toning effect. For best results the technique is administered frequently and for a number of minutes during each session.

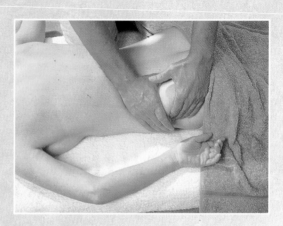

1 *This technique follows crisscross effleurage.* Kneeling at the side of the recipient, reach over to the opposite side of the lower back to carry out the petrissage. Start with the fingers of one hand on the outer part of the loin and the thumb of the second hand on the lower back muscles. Here, pressure is being applied with the fingers of the left hand against the thumb of the right.

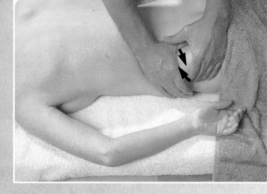

2 Lift up the tissues with the fingers of one hand as you gently push down with the thumb of the other hand.

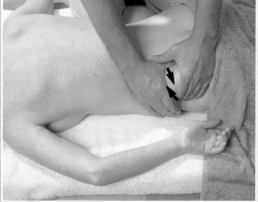

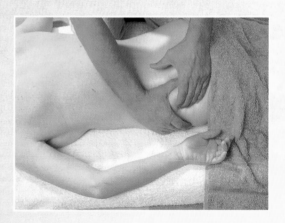

3 After squeezing the tissues, slide the hands off and release the pressure.

Repeat technique

CRISS-CROSS
EFFLEURAGE
See page 60
•
Followed by
PETRISSAGE

4 Repeat the movement a few times with the fingers of each hand alternately starting on the outer loin area. Here, the pressure is being applied between the fingers of the right hand against the thumb of the left. This petrissage technique can also be applied to the buttock muscles.

PERCUSSIVE MOVEMENTS: CUPPING

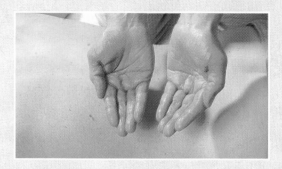

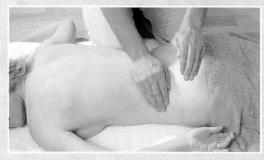

1 Suspend the hands just above the area to be worked on. Cup each hand by curving the palm and fingers, and tighten the whole hand as if you are holding a tennis ball (with the hand held palm-side down and without closing the fingers). The cupped hand strikes the tissues, making a deep sound, as the arm bends from the elbow.

2 One hand strikes as the other is lifted off. Continue with this alternating cupping of the tissues for a few minutes.

Gentle percussive movements can be carried out on the loins to help tone up the tissues, avoiding delicate and fragile areas like the lower rib cage, kidneys, and spine. Both little finger strikes and cupping are done, but with very little weight added. The buttocks, too, will benefit from these techniques, and the weight of the strokes can be slightly heavier in this area.

PERCUSSIVE MOVEMENTS: LITTLE FINGER STRIKE

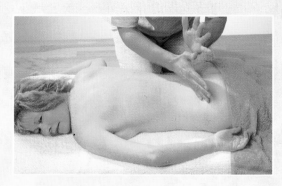

1 Hold the hands slightly above the area to be worked on, with the palms facing each other and the fingers apart. Bend each hand sideways from the wrist to strike the tissues with the little finger. No weight other than that of the hand itself is required. Ensure that the outside border of the palm of the hand does not strike the tissue karate-style.

2 Lift up the striking hand as the second hand comes down to percuss. Keep the hands very close to each other. They should rebound from the muscle – be careful not to hit it with a thud. Continue with this alternating striking at a leisurely pace for a few minutes. *Continue with lymph drainage.*

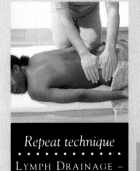

Repeat technique

LYMPH DRAINAGE –
LOIN AREA
See page 149
•
Followed by
CIRCULAR PALM
EFFLEURAGE – TO
THE ABDOMEN

PREGNANCY

7

THE ABDOMEN

The abdominal muscles run in two directions: one group runs vertically between the breastbone and the pubic bone; the second runs diagonally from the rib cage to the centre and from the pelvic bones to the centre of the abdomen. During pregnancy they are stretched considerably, along with the skin, and are likely to require a lot of toning up for some weeks after childbirth. To complement exercise, which is the obvious remedy, massage, especially toning up techniques like petrissage, can be used very effectively.

PETRISSAGE – OUTER ABDOMINAL MUSCLES

Work on the muscles situated between the lower rib cage and the rim of the pelvis, commonly referred to as the hip.

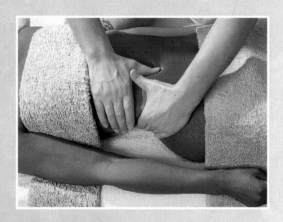

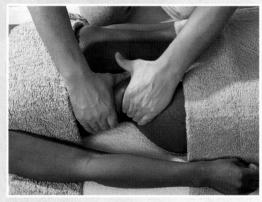

1 *This technique follows circular palm effleurage.* Position yourself on one side of the recipient and reach over to the opposite side of her abdomen. Place one hand round the abdomen towards the back, and place the second hand more to the front.

2 Use the fingers of one hand and the thumb of the second hand to lift and squeeze the tissues. Keep the thumb flat so as not to exert too much pressure. Release the tissues after a gentle squeeze.

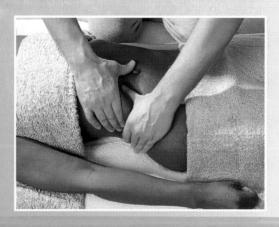

3 Continue to slide the hands so the starting positions have been reversed and repeat the lifting and squeezing movement. Repeat the whole stroke several times.

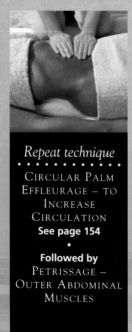

Repeat technique

CIRCULAR PALM
EFFLEURAGE – TO
INCREASE
CIRCULATION
See page 154

Followed by
PETRISSAGE –
OUTER ABDOMINAL
MUSCLES

PETRISSAGE – CENTRAL ABDOMINAL MUSCLES

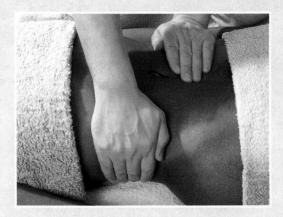 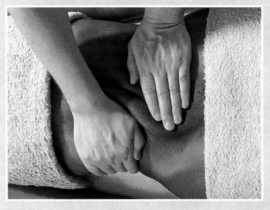

To ensure that the abdominal muscles are relaxed the recipients' hands should be at the side of her body or on her chest.

1 Place the hands on each side of the abdomen. Contact is with the palm and fingers. Apply a little pressure.

2 Move the hands towards the centre to gently lift up and squeeze the central abdominal muscles. Adjust the pressure to enable you to lift the tissues.

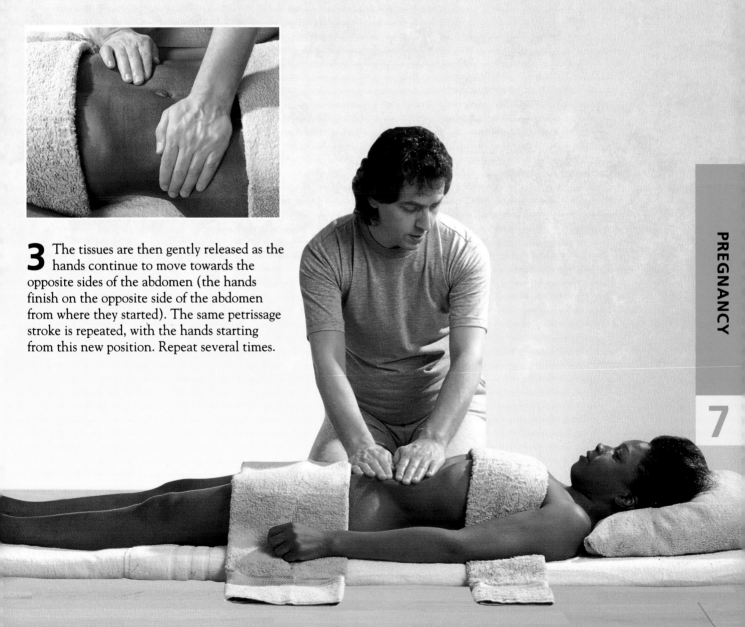

3 The tissues are then gently released as the hands continue to move towards the opposite sides of the abdomen (the hands finish on the opposite side of the abdomen from where they started). The same petrissage stroke is repeated, with the hands starting from this new position. Repeat several times.

LYMPH DRAINAGE –
ABDOMINAL TISSUES

This technique is very similar to that described on page 119 for lymph drainage during pregnancy. Very light effleurage to assist with the drainage is carried out from the level of the navel towards the groin, and from the same level of the navel towards the chest. As with other areas, any excessive or systemic fluid retention may need the attention of a doctor.

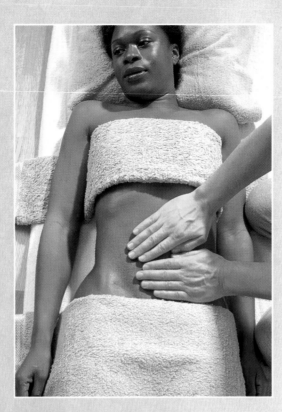

1 Position yourself to the side of the recipient. Place your hands next to each other in the centre of the abdomen with the fingers pointing away from you. Effleurage from the navel towards the groin on the opposite side, using very light pressure (the weight of the hand only). When the hands reach the far side, lift them off and return to the starting position. Repeat several times.

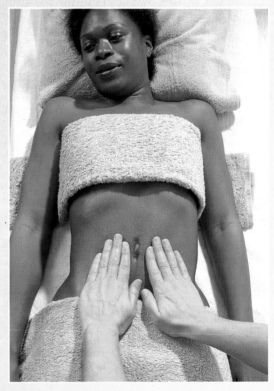

2 Place the hands next to each other in the centre of the abdomen but with the fingers pointing towards the chest. Keeping contact with all of the palm and fingers, effleurage upwards towards the chest. Use the same kind of pressure as in the previous stroke. When you reach a comfortable position on the chest lift off your hands and return to the starting position to repeat the movement several times.

SELF-ADMINISTERED MASSAGE

. . . .

The abdominal and thigh massage techniques can be carried out as self-administered movements in addition to (or in place of) the administered ones.

. . . .

PETRISSAGE – ABDOMINAL MUSCLES

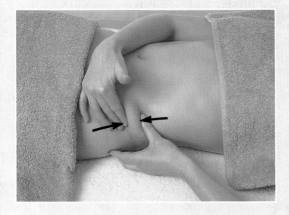

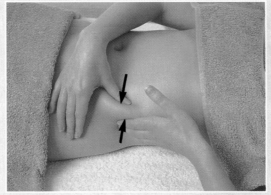

Lie on your back but prop yourself up on a couple of pillows. Bend your knees and support them on cushions.

1 Place both hands close together on one side of the abdomen to petrissage the outer muscles. The technique entails the lifting and squeezing of the tissues between the fingers of one hand and the thumb of the other. Release the tissues after the squeezing is applied (the same as the administered method).

2 Position the hands so as to repeat the lifting and squeezing. Continue for a few minutes. Apply the same stroke on the other side. Move the hands to the central area and repeat the technique on the central abdominal muscles.

. . . .

REPEAT TECHNIQUES

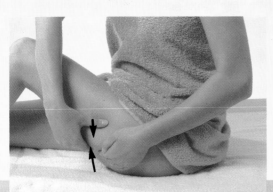

Repeat technique
. . . .
PETRISSAGE
See page 152
•
Followed by PERCUSSIVE MOVEMENTS

Repeat technique
. . . .
PERCUSSIVE MOVEMENTS
See page 153
•
This ends the sequence

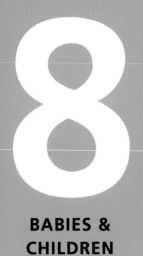

MASSAGE FOR BABIES AND CHILDREN

. . . .

Massaging a baby helps with the circulation and enhances body functions but even more important it provides you and your baby with some very enjoyable moments. Massaging a child is no different to massaging an adult. Children are as susceptible to tension, muscle aches and anxiety, and the objectives and benefits of the massage are therefore the same. Techniques, too, are very similar, except that the pressure reduces to suit the size of the muscles.

Baby massage is probably as instinctive as breast-feeding. It is as natural for the mother to give the massage as it is for the baby to receive it, though the father too can and should share this experience. Some movements are better done with the baby on your lap, others with him or her lying on a table. There are a great number of variations to the movements shown in the following pages. I suggest, therefore, that in addition to the techniques illustrated you use whatever seems obvious and natural. For example, although it is not demonstrated here, you can massage the baby as you hold him or her in your arms.

MASSAGE OILS

Lavender and camomile are the only two essential oils suitable for babies and even then they should be used in very small amounts, no more than one or two drops at a time. Lavender, for example, helps to promote sleep. A single drop is sufficient, put on a tissue nearby or on the cot sheet or pyjamas. Alternatively you can add it to the massage oil. Camomile or lavender can be used to massage the baby's tummy in cases of colic. Use one drop in an egg cup full of warmed up vegetable oil such as almond or soya. Massage this same mixture round the ear to ease earaches associated with teething or colds. Add a drop or two of camomile or lavender in the baby's bath to prevent nappy-rash.

Essential oils can irritate the eyes of both adults and babies alike. If you put any in a baby's bath be careful not to let your fingers, or the baby's, touch the eyes after they have been in the water.

MASSAGE FOR CHILDREN

Some children are too impatient to receive a full massage but are quite happy to accept a back and shoulder massage while sitting in front of you on the floor. The muscles of the legs and feet benefit tremendously from a soothing down massage after the running about children do.

MASSAGE OILS

As with babies the most common essential oils used are camomile and lavender. They are used in very small dosages, only about a two per cent mixture with a vegetable oil base.

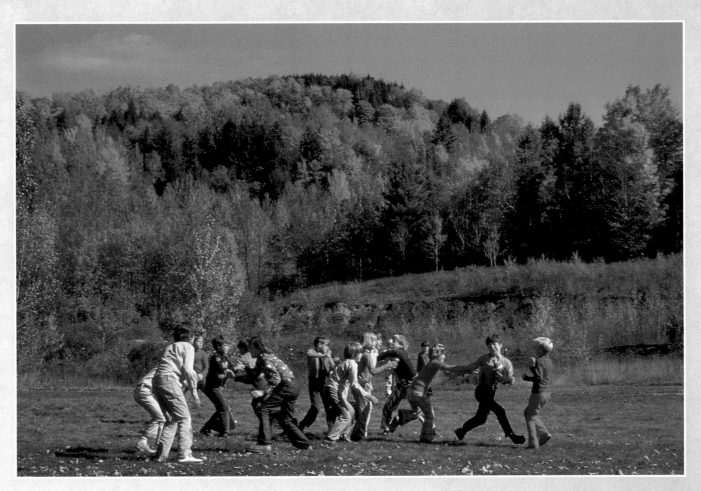

Playing and running around can result in muscle soreness, bruising and even slight injury. Children will benefit from regular massage.

BABIES **On your lap** ROUTINE ONE	BABIES **On a table** ROUTINE TWO	CHILDREN **Sitting** ROUTINE ONE
Circular effleurage – abdomen • **Effleurage – abdomen, chest and arms** • **Effleurage – front of leg** • **Effleurage – back** • **Effleurage – neck** • **Effleurage – back of the leg** • **Finger and thumb effleurage – spine** • **Gentle vibrations – back**	**Effleurage – abdomen, chest and arms** • **Effleurage – leg** • **Effleurage – both legs together** • **Effleurage – foot** • **Effleurage – hand** • **Effleurage – back**	**Palm effleurage – neck and shoulders** • **Thumb effleurage – shoulder muscles** • **Pick-up effleurage – neck muscles**

Lying

Palm effleurage – back
•
Palm effleurage – leg
•
Compressing effleurage – foot
•
Thumb effleurage – sole of foot

MASSAGING THE BABY ON YOUR LAP

. . . .

Lie the baby on your lap, with one hand supporting him or her. Use the other hand to effleurage in different directions. There is no need to apply any pressure with any of these techniques.

. . . .

CIRCULAR EFFLEURAGE – ABDOMEN

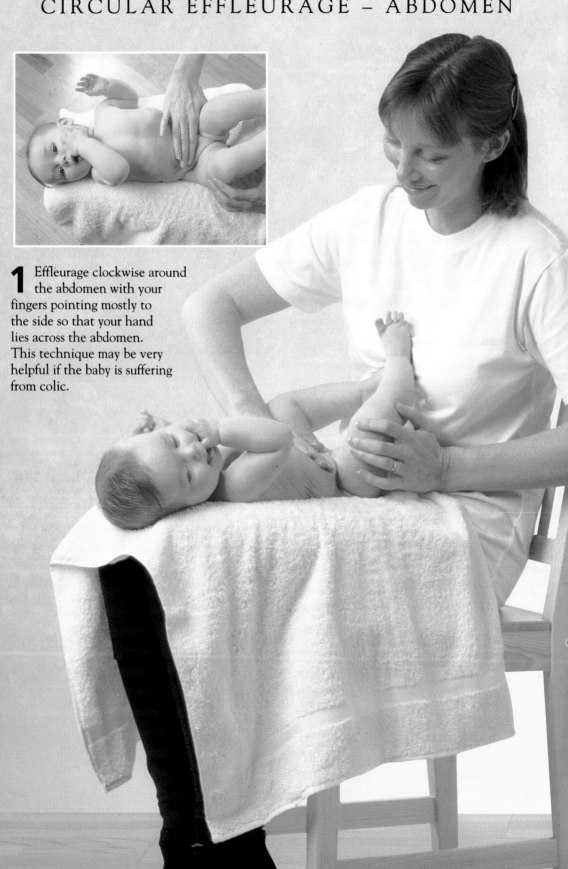

1 Effleurage clockwise around the abdomen with your fingers pointing mostly to the side so that your hand lies across the abdomen. This technique may be very helpful if the baby is suffering from colic.

EFFLEURAGE – ABDOMEN, CHEST AND ARMS

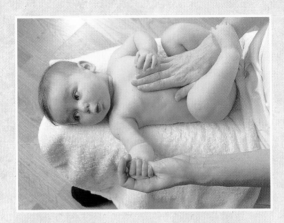 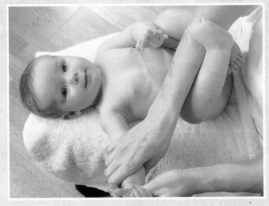

1 Place the hand on the abdomen with the fingers pointing away from you. Effleurage from the abdomen upwards towards the head and outwards towards the arm.

2 Continue by encircling the arm with the whole hand and effleuraging up the arm to the fingers.

EFFLEURAGE – FRONT OF LEG

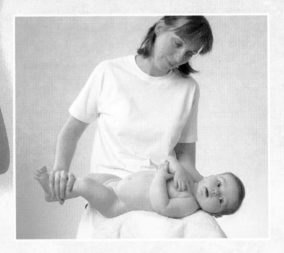 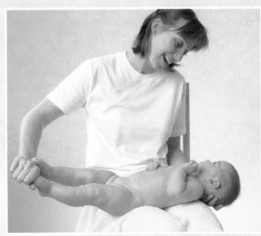

1 The hand encircles the leg at the thigh.

2 Effleurage the whole leg, adding a gentle squeeze, all the way to the toes. Repeat the massage on the other leg.

EFFLEURAGE – BACK OF NECK

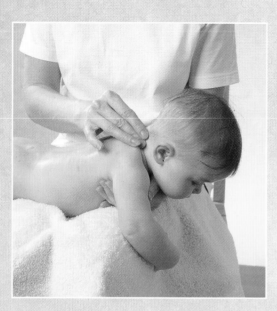

1 Place the fingers on one side of the neck and the thumb on the other side. Gently squeeze the neck between the fingers and thumb. While applying this very gentle squeeze let the neck slip away from your grip by sliding the hand upwards. The stroke can be combined with the back masage movement, carried out when the hands reach the top of the back.

EFFLEURAGE TO THE BACK

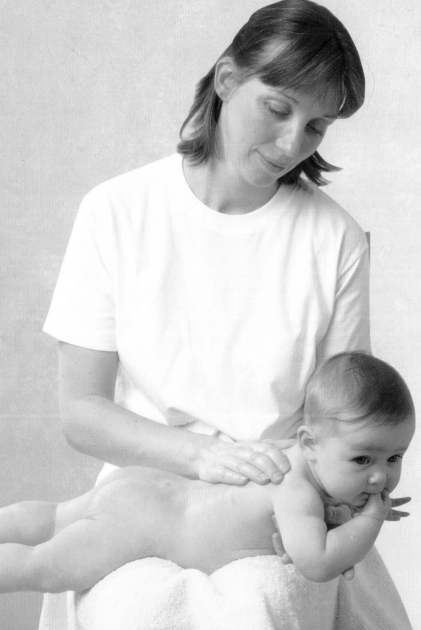

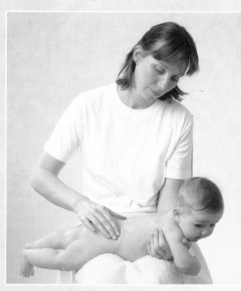

1 The baby is lying on his or her front across your lap. Place one hand at the lower end of the back, more or less on the buttocks. The hand is placed across the back with the fingers pointing away from you or along the back with the fingers pointing towards the head.

2 Effleurage by running the hand upwards towards the neck. Do not apply a lot of pressure and keep your hand very relaxed so as not to crease the baby's skin too much. When you reach the top of the back you can carry out the neck massage before returning to the buttocks to repeat the stroke.

EFFLEURAGE – BACK OF LEG

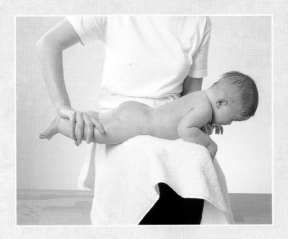

1 Effleurage down the leg with your hand, applying a gentle squeeze at the same time. Include the ankle and the whole foot right down to the toes. Repeat the massage on the other leg.

FINGER AND THUMB EFFLEURAGE – SPINE

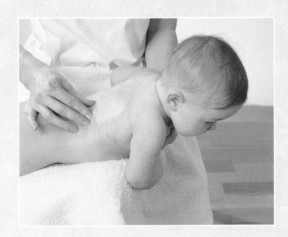

1 Use the first or middle finger and the thumb to apply a little pressure on each side of the spine. Starting at the base of the spine as far down as the buttocks, slide the fingers all the way up to the top of the neck.

GENTLE VIBRATIONS – BACK

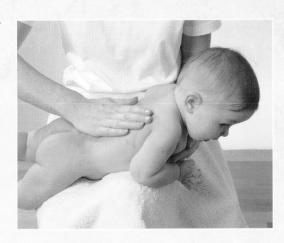

1 Place the flat hand on the small of the baby's back and gently vibrate for a few seconds.

MASSAGING THE BABY ON A TABLE

It may feel safer to massage the baby on the table instead of on your lap if he or she tends to wiggle about a lot.

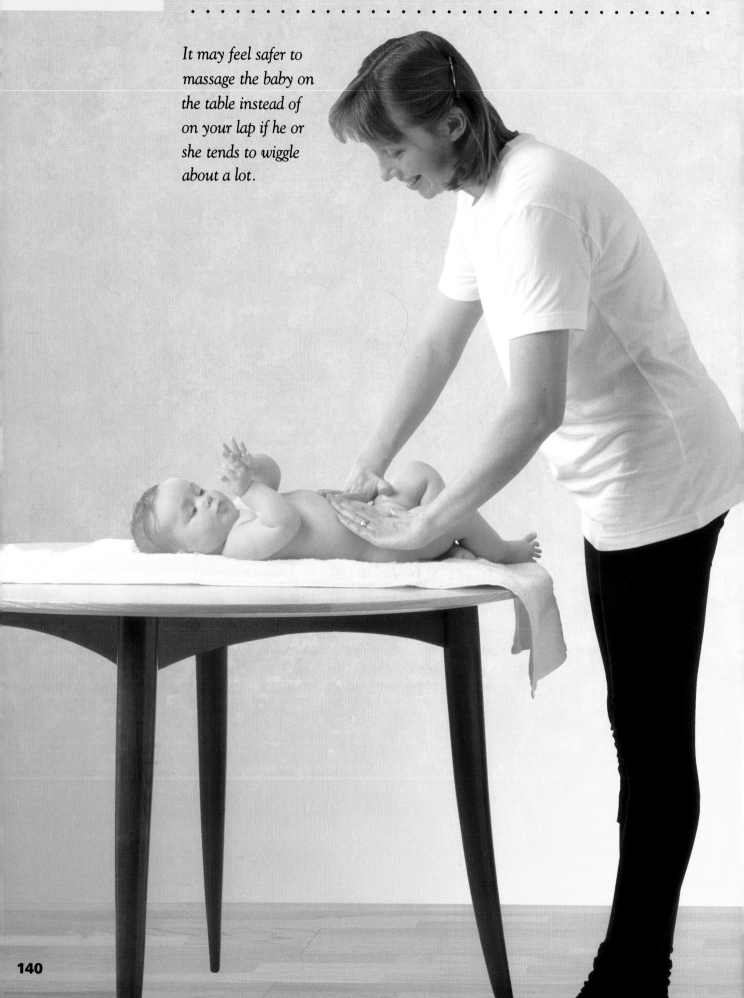

EFFLEURAGE – ABDOMEN, CHEST AND ARMS

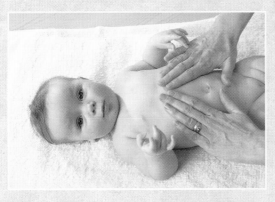 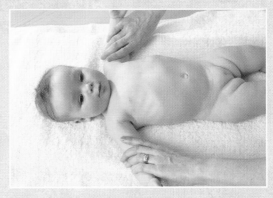

1 Lie baby on the table face upwards. Place both hands on the centre of the abdomen, with the fingers pointing towards each other. Effleurage up to the chest with both hands.

2 Then your hands separate, each hand effleurages an arm, working upwards to the fingers.

EFFLEURAGE – LEG

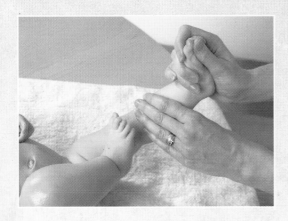

1 Hold one foot with one hand, and with the other effleurage the same leg starting at the ankle and finishing at the upper thigh. Repeat once or twice, and then repeat on the other leg.

EFFLEURAGE – BOTH LEGS TOGETHER

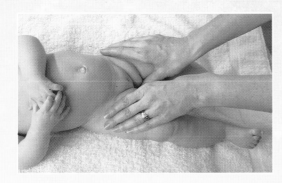 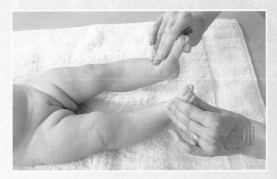

1 Effleurage both legs together with the hands applying a gentle squeeze as they move from the upper thigh to the foot.

2 Continue the stroke to include the toes.

THUMB EFFLEURAGE – FOOT

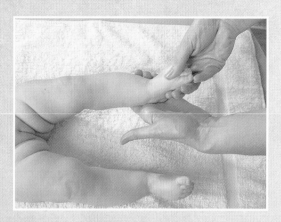 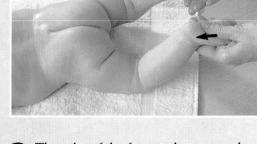

1 Massage the foot and toes by placing your thumb on the top of the foot and your fingers underneath. Start at the ankle and finish at the toes. You can also gently squeeze the whole foot with your hands in this position.

2 The soles of the feet can be massaged with the thumbs if the baby lies face down.

THUMB EFFLEURAGE – HAND

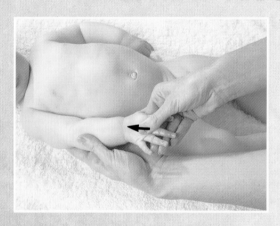

1 Massage each hand with the thumbs and fingers in a similar manner to the foot.

EFFLEURAGE – BACK

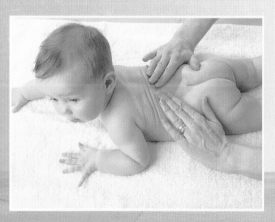

1 With the baby lying on his or her tummy, effleurage the back in the same way as when he or she is lying on your lap. One or both hands may be used.

MASSAGE FOR CHILDREN

The techniques illustrated in this position are equally suited to an adult.

PALM EFFLEURAGE –
NECK AND SHOULDERS

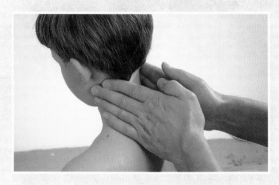

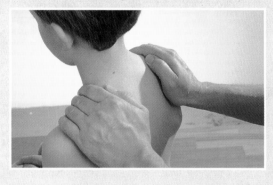

You may want to support the back of the child against your knees with a cushion used in between as padding.

1 The recipient sits in front of you on the floor or on a stool. Using one hand on each side, effleurage from the top of the neck down to the shoulders.

2 Cup the hands as you go over the shoulders.

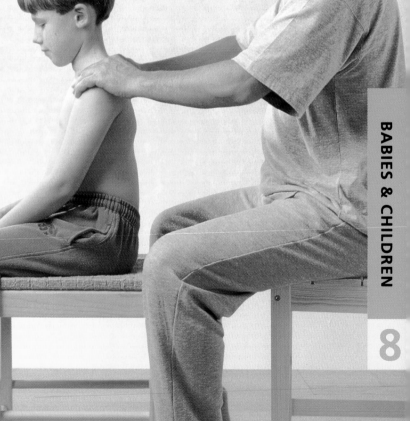

3 Finish the stroke at the top of the arms. Return the hands to the first position and repeat. It may be easier to do this movement with one hand effleuraging one side at a time. The recipient can sit slightly more to the side in this case.

THUMB EFFLEURAGE – SHOULDER MUSCLES

Work a little more deeply into the upper back and shoulder muscles using the thumb.

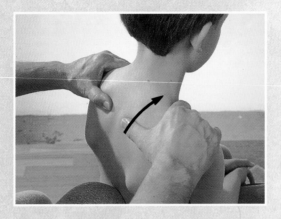

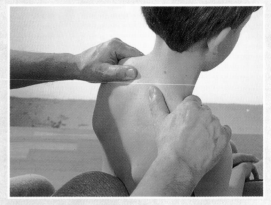

1 Placing a hand on each shoulder, start the stroke with the thumbs in between the spine and the shoulder blade, and the fingers placed on top of the shoulder. Press into the tissues as your thumbs travel towards your fingers.

2 When you get to the top of the shoulders ease off the pressure so as not to pinch the skin. Repeat several times.

PICK-UP EFFLEURAGE – NECK AND SHOULDERS

You may find it easier to carry out this movement if the recipient sits slightly sideways.

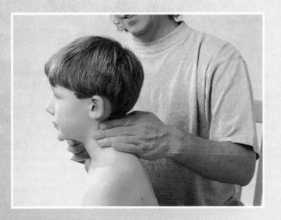

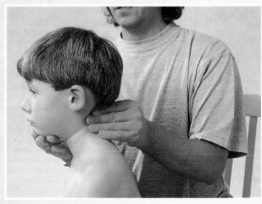

1 The recipient sits slightly turned to the side. Support the chin with one hand. The second hand is placed at the back of the neck with the thumb on one side and the fingers on the other side of the neck. Gently squeeze the muscles of the neck between the fingers and the thumb, taking care not to pinch the skin.

2 Hold on to the squeeze and gently pull the tissues away from the spine. Let your fingers slide off to release the hold. Repeat a few times.

PALM EFFLEURAGE – BACK

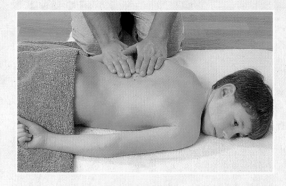

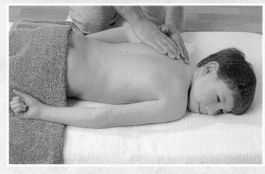

Position yourself beside the recipient, at about his or her waist level. The effleurage involves two strokes, one on the side of the trunk nearest to you and the other on the far side. If you find it difficult to reach the far side, move round and work on one side at a time.

1 Place your hands beside the spine on the side nearest to you with the fingers pointing towards the opposite side. Start at the lower back and effleurage upwards towards the shoulder, the hands travelling on the same side of the spine nearest to you.

2 Continue the movement over the shoulder and down the outside of the trunk nearest to you.

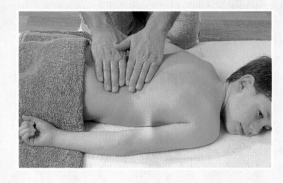

3 Place your hands on the lower back again but beside the spine on the side furthest away from you.

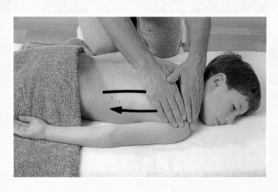

4 Repeat the stroke on that side of the spine including the opposite shoulder and outer part of the trunk. This completes the whole movement. Repeat several times.

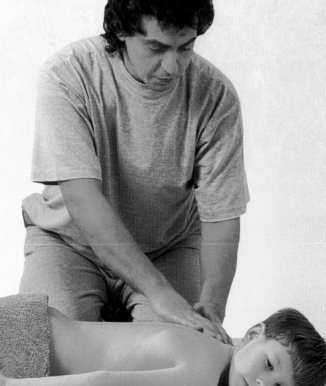

PALM EFFLEURAGE – LEG

Palm effleurage can be applied to the back, as well as the front of the leg.

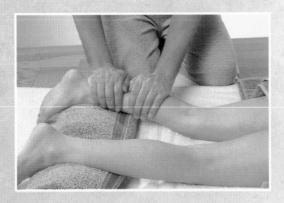

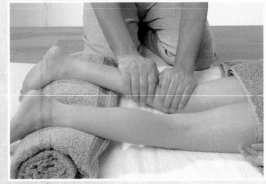

1 The recipient lies face down. Place your hands on top of the leg nearest to you, with the fingers pointing away from you.

2 Effleurage with both hands travelling together from the ankle to the upper thigh. Apply a little pressure and give a gentle squeeze as you move upwards with the hands but ease off over the back of the knee. With a very light stroke return to the ankle for the movement to be repeated.

Massage the other leg in the same manner; and the front of the legs, following the same procedure and technique as for the back of the legs (without putting pressure on the shin bone).

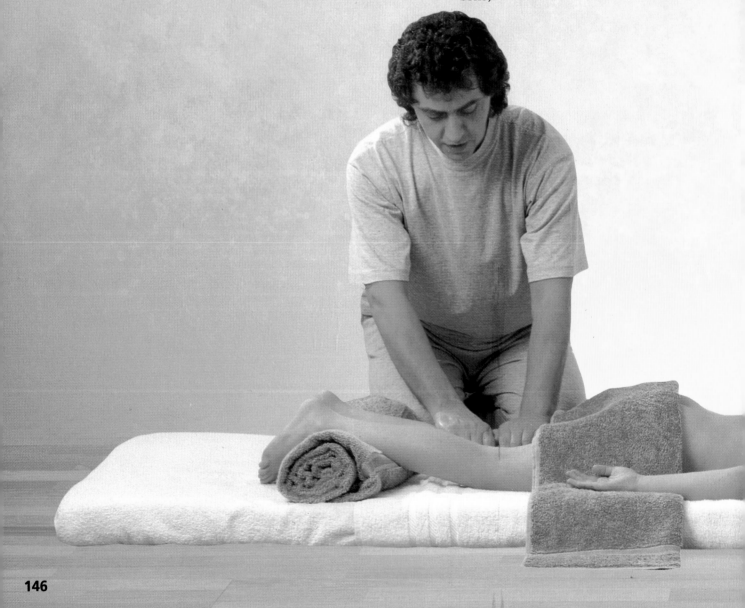

COMPRESSING EFFLEURAGE – FOOT

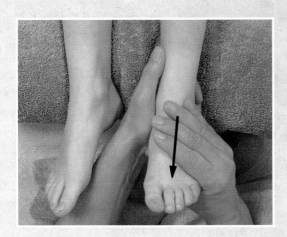

1 Rest the recipient's foot on a cushion or rolled-up towel in front of you, with him or her lying face upwards. Position your fingers across the top of the foot and your thumb across the sole. Compress the foot gently between the fingers and thumb as you slide the hand from the heel to the toes. Repeat several times using the same hand, or alternate hands.

You can also carry out this movement with the recipient's foot resting on your lap as you sit on the floor.

THUMB EFFLEURAGE – SOLE OF FOOT

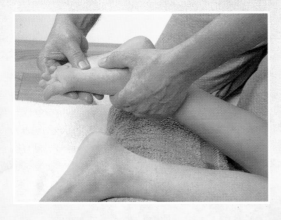

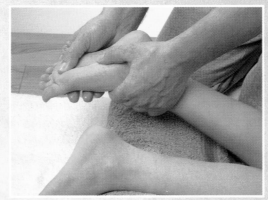

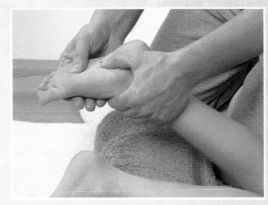

If the feet are dry, apply plenty of oil to carry out this movement. Use positive pressure to ensure that the strokes are not ticklish to the recipient.

1 The recipient lies face downwards with the knee bent so the foot is lifted up and resting on your hands.

2 Use one or alternate thumbs to massage the sole of the foot.

3 The strokes can be done as a series of small semi-circles or as short, straight movements.

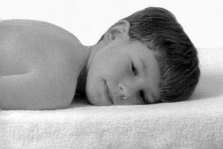

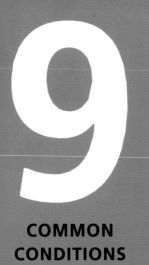

COMMON CONDITIONS

Cellulite, PMT and digestion are further examples where massage can be applied for therapeutic effect. In some cases, it may be necessary to combine administered and self-administered techniques with other methods of treatment. The massage routines are also equally effective as a preventative measure.

PRE-MENSTRUAL TENSION

The pre-menstrual syndrome (PMT) is a very delicate and intricate malady. It is not within the scope of this book to cover the subject in detail, but rather to refer to some aspects of it in relation to massage. A number of symptoms are associated with the condition and there are perhaps an equal number of approaches to its treatment. The more naturopathic of these include dietary changes and supplementation, such as eliminating sugars, starches and refined food from the diet and reducing or eliminating stimulants like coffee, tea and alcohol. Supplements include evening primrose oil and vitamins B6 and B12. Fluid retention and abdominal cramps are among the physical symptoms of PMT; emotional manifestations include irritability and anxiety. Massage is very beneficial in dealing with some of these manifestations.

MASSAGE OILS

. . . .

For fluid retention
Geranium • Rosemary

For depression and irritability
Bergamot • Camomile • Rose

For anxiety
**Bergamot • Camomile
• Clary sage • Frankincense
• Jasmine • Marjoram • Melissa
• Neroli • Rose • Sandalwood
• Ylang-ylang**

effleurage strokes are carried out to the outer aspect of the breast towards the armpit. The upper region is drained in this manner towards the collar bone and the inner area is drained towards the breastbone.

FLUID RETENTION

The extent of the fluid build-up can vary from month to month and from person to person. If it is excessive the woman may require medical treatment, or treatment by a complementary therapist who specializes in manual lymph drainage or reflex zone therapy. If it is not severe enough for this, then the massage techniques for lymph drainage shown in previous chapters can be applied.

Although it is not shown in this book, breast tissue benefits significantly from lymph drainage techniques. Light

RELAXING MASSAGE

Most massage techniques, apart from the toning-up ones, are relaxing, so the majority of them can be used to reduce anxiety or tension. The woman receiving

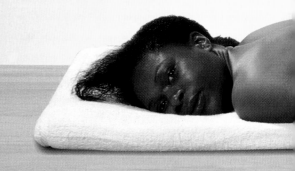

the massage may have her own preferences but massage to the back and the face is particularly worthwhile. Take extra care when massaging the stomach and the breast tissue because these can be, in some cases, very sensitive and tender. Abdominal and uterine cramps usually respond well to massage and consequently any related tenderness should ease off gradually. Massage to these areas may have to be omitted in cases of extreme soreness.

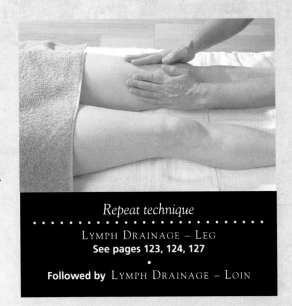

Repeat technique

· ·

LYMPH DRAINAGE – LEG
See pages 123, 124, 127
·
Followed by LYMPH DRAINAGE – LOIN

· ·

LYMPH DRAINAGE – LOIN AREA

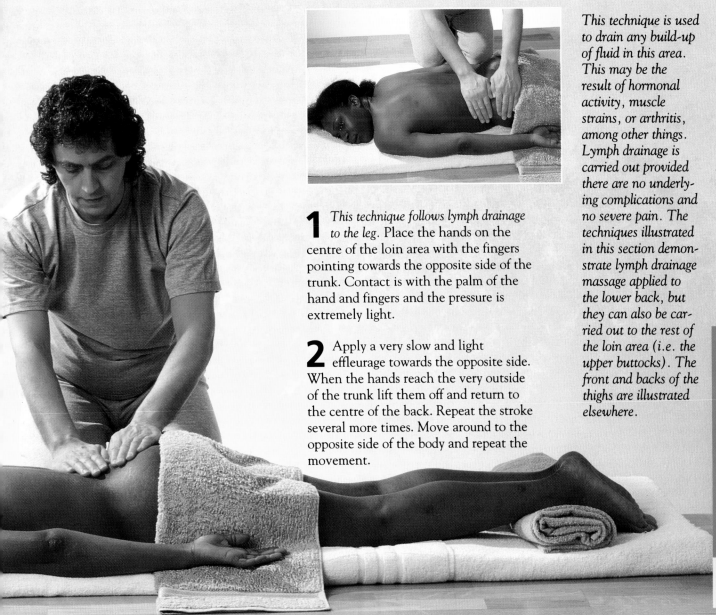

1 *This technique follows lymph drainage to the leg.* Place the hands on the centre of the loin area with the fingers pointing towards the opposite side of the trunk. Contact is with the palm of the hand and fingers and the pressure is extremely light.

2 Apply a very slow and light effleurage towards the opposite side. When the hands reach the very outside of the trunk lift them off and return to the centre of the back. Repeat the stroke several more times. Move around to the opposite side of the body and repeat the movement.

This technique is used to drain any build-up of fluid in this area. This may be the result of hormonal activity, muscle strains, or arthritis, among other things. Lymph drainage is carried out provided there are no underlying complications and no severe pain. The techniques illustrated in this section demonstrate lymph drainage massage applied to the lower back, but they can also be carried out to the rest of the loin area (i.e. the upper buttocks). The front and backs of the thighs are illustrated elsewhere.

REFLEX POINTS

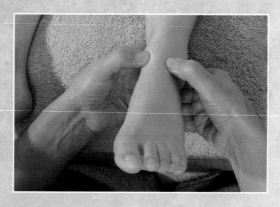

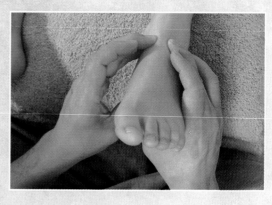

Pelvic lymphatics: The region between the outside and inside ankle bones reflexes the lymphatics (fluid draining system) around the pelvis. Massage using the thumbs or fingertips in this region, along the crease line.

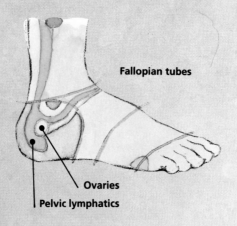

Fallopian tubes

Ovaries

Pelvic lymphatics

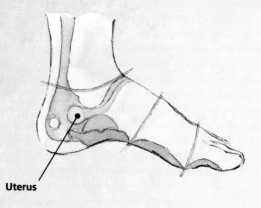

Uterus

Fallopian tubes: Reflex points for the fallopian tubes are found in the central area along the same line as the pelvic lymphatics.

Ovaries and uterus: Reflex points for these areas are found just below the outside and the inside ankle bones. They can be massaged gently with the thumb.

Solar plexus: See page 29.

ACUPRESSURE POINTS

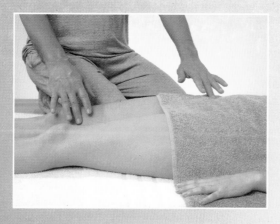

Acupressure points for PMT. These two points are treated together.

Point SP10: This point is located on the inside of the thigh. Recognized by its tenderness, it is found three fingers' width above the top of the knee.

Point SP13: To find this point, imagine a line running between the outer pelvic bone and the pubic bone, along the crease formed by the top of the thigh and the pelvis. Find the centre of this line: the point is two fingers' width above.

CELLULITE

Cellulite is a hardening of the fat cells. It is sometimes wrongly referred to as cellulitis, which is inflammation of tissues just below the skin, and it is associated with hormonal activity in women. Cellulite is a collection of fibrous bags made from collagen fibres which form around fat cells, trapping inside them fluid and toxins. When this happens to great numbers of fat cells the overall effect is a thickening and hardening of the tissues and a bumpy texture skin.

Apart from the hormones causing fluid retention, the problem also arises from wrong diet, which can contribute to an increase in toxins and fat cells; and from bad circulation, which can be due to lack of exercise. All of these factors need

to be addressed if cellulite is to be reduced or prevented. Massage is certainly very effective in improving the circulation, including that of lymph, and it also keeps the tissues toned up.

MASSAGE OILS

To assist circulation
Lemon • Camomile • Cypress • Black pepper • Juniper • Marjoram

To assist lymph drainage
Fennel • Geranium • Juniper • Rosemary

To reduce toxins
Fennel • Juniper • Garlic • Rose

SELF-ADMINISTERED SKIN BRUSHING

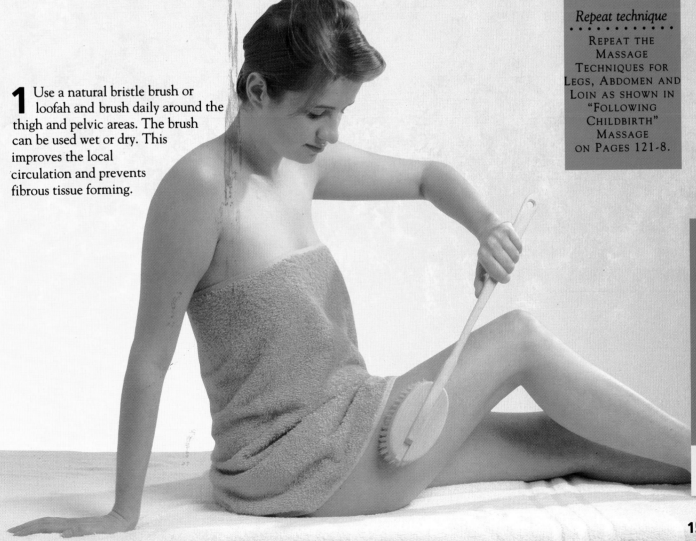

1 Use a natural bristle brush or loofah and brush daily around the thigh and pelvic areas. The brush can be used wet or dry. This improves the local circulation and prevents fibrous tissue forming.

Repeat technique

REPEAT THE MASSAGE TECHNIQUES FOR LEGS, ABDOMEN AND LOIN AS SHOWN IN "FOLLOWING CHILDBIRTH" MASSAGE ON PAGES 121-8.

COMMON CONDITIONS

9

151

PETRISSAGE – THIGH MUSCLES:
SELF-ADMINISTERED

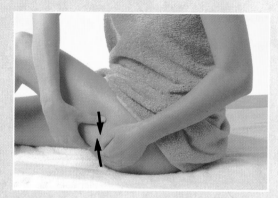

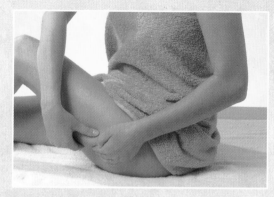

1 Sit on the floor. The petrissage is done by using the fingers of one hand and the thumb of the other to work on the muscles of the thigh. The heel of the hand can be used instead of the thumb.

2 Apply pressure between the two hands to compress and lift the muscles, adding a gentle twist at the same time. Avoid pinching the skin. Relax the grip and so release the muscles and tissues.

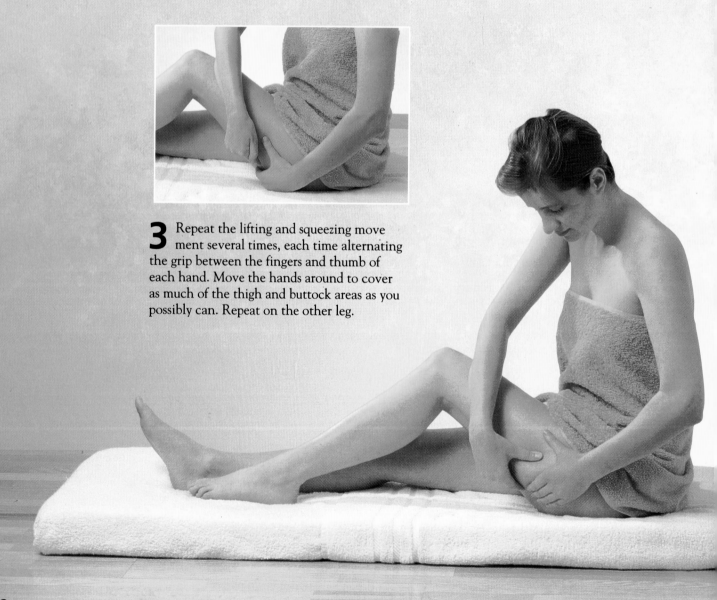

3 Repeat the lifting and squeezing move ment several times, each time alternating the grip between the fingers and thumb of each hand. Move the hands around to cover as much of the thigh and buttock areas as you possibly can. Repeat on the other leg.

PERCUSSIVE MOVEMENTS – THIGH MUSCLES: SELF-ADMINISTERED

While sitting on the floor use the percussive strokes to tone up the thigh muscles. Adjust your posture to find a comfortable position. It is also possible for these strokes to be done while sitting on a chair.

LITTLE FINGER STRIKE

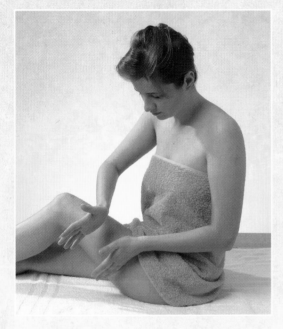

1 Sit on the floor with your legs straight or slightly bent at the knees and supported by a cushion. Reach to the outer side of the thigh and percuss the tissues with the little finger of each hand. Alternate the hands so that as one hand is striking the other one is lifting off.

2 Change the position of the hands to cover as much of the region as possible.

CUPPING

1 Still in the same sitting position, use the cupped hands to percuss the areas, as in the previous stroke. Cup the hands by curving the palm and fingers slightly, keep the fingers together and the whole hand slightly stiff.

2 Alternate the striking with each hand and move them around to cover as much of the area as possible.

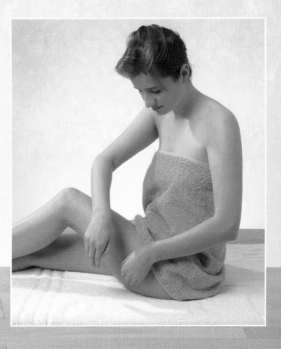

DIGESTION

The chief organs concerned with digestion are the stomach and intestines, and this is where common problems relating to digestion are experienced. More serious but less frequent problems range from diarrhoea, ulcers and appendicitis to diverticulitis and cancer. Needless to say their treatment is a matter for the medical profession. Nonetheless, massage benefits the digestive system because it improves the circulation of the abdomen and, in turn, the function of the digestive organs. Some techniques are specific, like massage to the colon. Most beneficial, however, is the relaxation aspect of massage which has an indirect effect on the whole digestive system.

MASSAGE OILS

For constipation
Marjoram • Rosemary

To reduce muscle spasm like that associated with indigestion or colic
Bergamot • Camomile • Clary Sage • Fennel • Melissa • Neroli • Peppermint

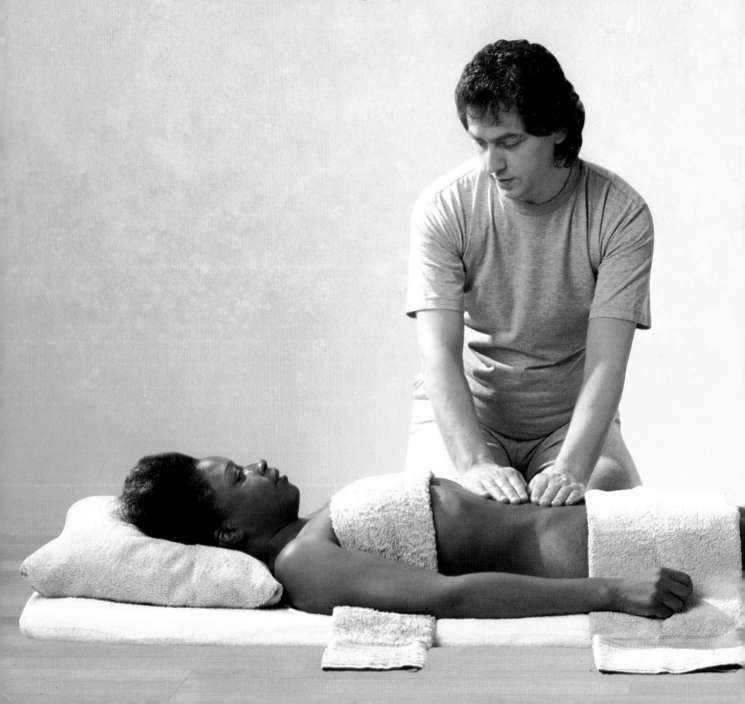

CIRCULAR PALM EFFLEURAGE – ABDOMEN

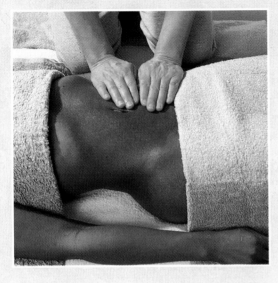

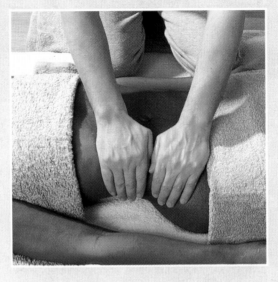

Palm effleurage is used to enhance the circulation and warm up the muscles. Pressure has to be very light to start with and then increased gradually without causing any discomfort.

1 Place the hands on the side of the abdomen nearest to you. Make contact with the palm and fingers and keep the hands close together and very relaxed. The movement is administered clockwise round the abdomen

2 Start the clockwise effleurage by moving the hands towards the opposite side of the abdomen reaching as far across as possible.

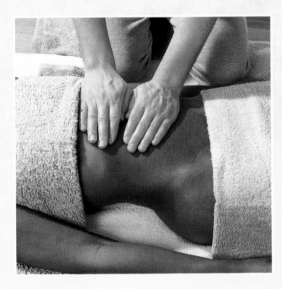

3 Continue the effleurage by moving the hands towards the centre and just below the rib cage. To complete the clockwise action, the hands continue to move to the side of the abdomen nearest to you. Repeat the whole movement several times.

Take care not to:

Massage the abdomen if any of the following are present:
•
ulcers, diverticulitis, Crohn's disease, chronic constipation diarrhoea, cancer, appendicitis, unexplained heat, inflammation, gallstones

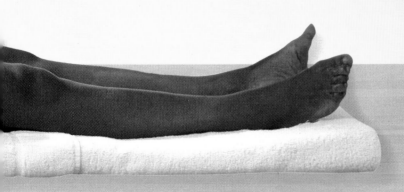

COMMON CONDITIONS

9

PALM EFFLEURAGE – COLON

The large intestine or colon is an inverted U shape, the first upright of which is the ascending colon running from the lower abdomen on the right to the bottom rib on the same side. The horizontal transverse colon then travels across from the right to the left side just below the rib cage. Completing the inverted U shape is the last part of the colon, which descends from the left lower rib down the left side of the abdomen towards the central pelvic area. Massage to the colon follows these three sections, the purpose being to aid movement of its contents. This requires sensitivity and patience as it can be tender to touch and it may take a little time to achieve the desired effect. Relaxing the recipient and the abdominal muscles should always precede this technique.

Take care not to:
· · · · · · · · · · ·

Massage the abdomen if any of the following conditions are suspected

·

diverticulitis, Crohn's disease, ulcers, cancer

·

any other serious disease or inflammatory condition

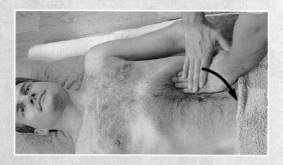

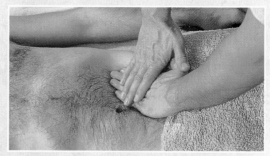

1 Position yourself on the left side of the recipient. Place the left hand just below the bottom of the left rib cage, with the fingers pointing towards the ribs. This hand feels the tissues and applies the stroke but not the pressure. Place the right hand on top and across the left hand, with the fingers pointing away from you. This hand applies the pressure.

2 Descending colon stroke. Adjusting the pressure as you move, effleurage down the left side of the abdomen towards the pelvic bone. Repeat several times.

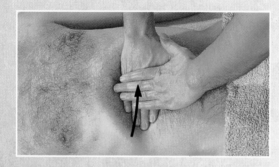

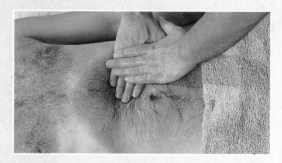

3 Transverse colon stroke. Position your right hand just below the bottom of the right rib cage with the fingers pointing away from you. This hand feels the tissues and applies the stroke but not the pressure. Place your left hand on top and across the right hand with the fingers pointing towards the head. This hand applies the pressure.

4 Effleurage with both hands in this position across the abdomen towards you. Repeat several times.

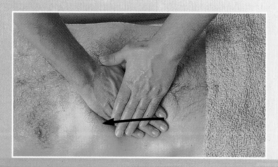

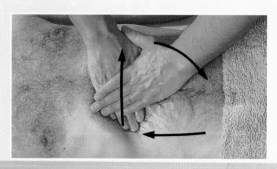

5 Ascending colon stroke. Place your right hand on the right side of the abdomen with the fingers pointing towards the pelvis. The tips of the fingers should be in line with the navel and not any lower. Put the left hand on top and across the right hand with the fingers pointing away from you.

6 Effleurage upwards to the bottom of the right rib cage. When you feel confident you can lengthen each stroke: Descending colon – a few times; transverse continuing on to the descending colon – a few times; ascending continuing to the transverse and to the descending colon – a few times.

REFLEX POINTS: COLON

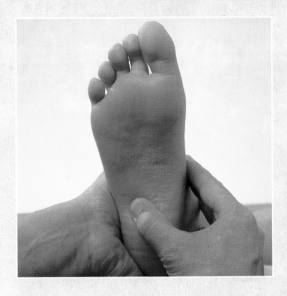

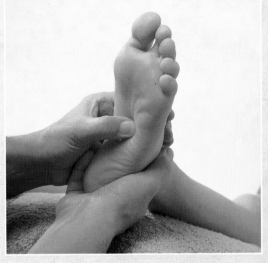

As with the colon massage, work on these reflex points by following the descending, transverse and finally the ascending colon sequence. As you apply the on/off pressure along these lines, ask the recipient for feedback on any pinprick type of pain. This will indicate a zone of reflex activity requiring treatment.

1 The reflex area on the foot relating to the colon follows the same U shape as the massage. The ascending colon is on the right foot. Also on the right foot is half of the transverse colon.

2 The other half of the transverse colon and the descending colon are on the left foot.

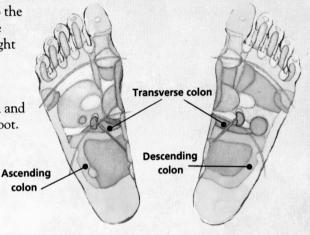

Transverse colon

Ascending colon

Descending colon

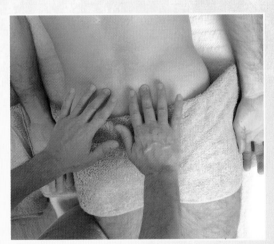

Repeat technique
REFLEX MASSAGE TO THE SOLAR PLEXUS
See page 29
•
Followed by
ACUPRESSURE POINTS

ACUPRESSURE POINTS

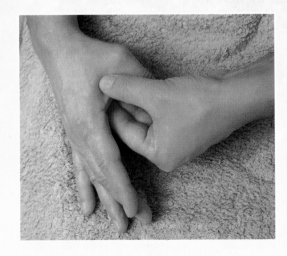

Point LI 4: Hoku point (LI 4). This point is located in the web between the thumb and index finger. Press gently for a few seconds with your thumb. This point should not be stimulated during pregnancy.

Point B48: Find this point by locating the two "dimples" on each side of the spine at the base (sacrum) where it meets the top of the pelvic bones (iliac crests). Apply light pressure to the points on the left and right sides simultaneously.

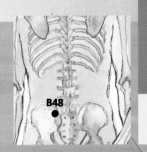

B48

COMMON CONDITIONS

9

. . . .

ACKNOWLEDGMENTS

The author would like to dedicate this book to Phyllis Evans in appreciation for her tremendous help and
support.

All photography by Paul Forrester with the exception of the following:
page 8 Wellcome Institute Library, London; pages 82, 135 Image Bank.

Quarto would like to thank Neals Yard Remedies, London for loaning oil bottles for photography.

Quarto would especially like to thank the models: Stephen Atkinson, Dominic Chapman, Angelo Garcia,
Kate and Lara Havelock, Hazel Jackman, Sarah Lambie, Maureen Newman, Theresa Nicolson, Alison
Pollock, Eamonn Shanahan, Richard Varcoe and Beverly Williamson.

Index by Dorothy Frame